CHANGING THE RULES

A CLIENT-DIRECTED APPROACH
TO THERAPY

THE GUILFORD FAMILY THERAPY SERIES
Alan S. Gurman, *Editor*

Recent volumes

CHANGING THE RULES: A CLIENT-DIRECTED APPROACH
TO THERAPY
Barry L. Duncan, Andrew D. Solovey, and Gregory S. Rusk

TRANSGENERATIONAL FAMILY THERAPIES
Laura Giat Roberto

THE INTIMACY PARADOX: PERSONAL AUTHORITY
IN THE FAMILY SYSTEM
Donald S. Williamson

HUSBANDS, WIVES, AND LOVERS: THE EMOTIONAL SYSTEM
OF THE EXTRAMARITAL AFFAIR
David J. Moultrup

MEN IN THERAPY: THE CHALLENGE OF CHANGE
Richard L. Meth and Robert S. Pasick with Barry Gordon,
Jo Ann Allen, Larry B. Feldman, and Sylvia Gordon

FAMILY SYSTEMS IN MEDICINE
Christian N. Ramsey, Jr., *Editor*

NEGOTIATING PARENT–ADOLESCENT CONFLICT:
A BEHAVIORAL–FAMILY SYSTEMS APPROACH
Arthur L. Robin and Sharon L. Foster

FAMILY TRANSITIONS: CONTINUITY AND CHANGE
OVER THE LIFE CYCLE
Celia Jaes Falicov, *Editor*

FAMILIES AND LARGER SYSTEMS: A FAMILY THERAPIST'S GUIDE
THROUGH THE LABYRINTH
Evan Imber-Black

AFFECTIVE DISORDERS AND THE FAMILY:
ASSESSMENT AND TREATMENT
John F. Clarkin, Gretchen Haas, and Ira D. Glick, *Editors*

CHANGING THE RULES

A CLIENT-DIRECTED APPROACH

TO THERAPY

BARRY L. DUNCAN

ANDREW D. SOLOVEY

GREGORY S. RUSK

The Guilford Press

New York   London

Last digit is print number: 9 8 7 6 5 4 3 2 1

Cataloging-in-Publication Information

Duncan, Barry L.
    Changing the rules : a client-directed approach to therapy / Barry
L. Duncan, Andrew D. Solovey, Gregory S. Rusk.
      p. cm.   —   (The Guilford family therapy series)
    Includes bibliographical references and index.
    ISBN 0-89862-108-9
    1. Eclectic psychotherapy.   2. Client-centered psychotherapy.
3. Psychotherapy—Evaluation.   4. Psychotherapist and patient.
5. Psychotherapy—Philosophy   I. Solovey, Andrew D.   II. Rusk,
Gregory S.   III. Title.   IV. Series.
    [DNLM: 1. Nondirective Therapy.   WM 420 D911c]
RC489.E24D86   1992
616.89'14—dc20
DNLM/DLC
for Library of Congress   92-1550
                                     CIP

To our wives, Karen, Donna, and Mary,
and to our children,
Jesse, Matthew, Nick, Anne,
Steven, Joe, and Charlie.
We love you.

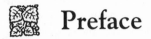 # Preface

MANY therapists discover the need to reassess their assumptions about their clinical practices after experience shatters the illusions provided by their chosen orientations. Consider the following vignettes:

Karen is a therapist in a community mental health center and is seeing Jim, a client who is suffering from seemingly inexplicable panic attacks and anxiety. She approaches her work as a therapist seriously and has continued to upgrade her skills and knowledge base since completing graduate school. She has always been impressed with the empirical support of behavioral approaches, but considers herself a strategically oriented therapist, largely because of an internship experience that followed a strategic model.

Given her orientation, Karen investigates Jim's coping style and his current solution attempts for addressing his problem. Karen employs relaxation techniques and symptom prescription to promote the acquisition of coping skills, as well as to bring the involuntary panic episodes under voluntary control. Jim's panic and anxiety do not diminish, and he reiterates a desire to know why the panic exists. Karen does not believe in the importance of knowing "why" and views such archaeological explorations as unhelpful digressions that only de-focus therapy from the presenting problem. Jim's anxiety does not abate, and he drops out of therapy.

Paul is a therapist in a juvenile-court diversion program and is seeing Kathy, a single parent whose son is in trouble for starting fires. Paul became disenchanted with individual approaches to therapy in graduate school and has been a strong advocate for a family/systems perspective ever since attending a workshop by a famous therapist from the Philadelphia Child Guidance Clinic. In that workshop, he observed a videotape example of an intervention with a family that also had a "fire starter." Impressed with the artful way in which the famous therapist handled the case, Paul followed that early experience with a commitment to learn as much as he could about structural family therapy, which included the completion of an externship training program.

Paul employed a variation of the famous therapist's intervention with the fire starter case, with limited results. He continued to work with Kathy and her son through a variety of distressful circumstances (e.g., death of Kathy's mother). From his orientation as a structural family therapist, Paul utilized in-session enactments to enable Kathy to establish proper boundaries and restore herself to an executive position within the family. He noted improvement, and it was clear to Paul that the restructuring of Kathy's relationship with her son, as well as her ex-husband, eliminated the need for the son's symptom. In the termination session, Paul asked what Kathy thought was most helpful to her. Kathy's response made no mention of any particular intervention; instead she identified what she appreciated the most was that Paul was "there" with her in her time of greatest need.

Mike is a therapist in private practice and is seeing Nancy, a client who is experiencing depression related to the recent breakup of her marriage. He has diligently pursued a neoanalytic orientation since a highly satisfactory training experience in graduate school. To further that pursuit, he continues a supervisory relationship with his mentor. Mike scrupulously attempts to provide the conditions necessary for Nancy to explore the historical antecedents to her current distress. He consciously works to enable a respectful space for Nancy's productions by giving very little verbally himself. From his theoretical perspective, he firmly believes that her productions are far more important than his and that his patient listening is conveying an ultimate form of respect.

Nancy becomes very frustrated with her lack of progress in therapy. Mike views her frustration as resistance and hypothesizes that she is struggling with the care and respect inherent in the therapeutic relationship. Mike interprets this hypothesized struggle as being related to events from Nancy's childhood. Nancy disagrees and shares her overall dissatisfaction with therapy. After much deliberation and consultation with his supervisor, Mike modifies his interactive style with Nancy. He begins to talk more and share more of himself; at times the sessions seem more "conversational" than therapeutic by the standards of his neoanalytic model. At termination, Nancy reports feeling significantly better and reveals that while she thought Mike too young at first, he seemed to have matured during the course of her therapy!

The vignettes of Karen, Paul, and Mike characterize the development of many therapists. Each was influenced by an early experience: Karen completed an internship that operated from a strategic orientation; Paul was strongly influenced by the work of a renowned structural family therapist; and Mike was supervised in graduate school from a neoanalytic perspective. Regardless of professional affiliation, many therapists share a similar history and are exposed to the inherent rightness of a given approach. We tend to view proponents of our chosen approaches as heroes/heroines and emulate them in the hope that our chosen orientations will provide definitive answers for the amelioration of human suffering.

All too soon, though, therapists are confronted with cases that do not seem to fit their chosen model's assumptions. Jim, Karen's client, desired to know "why" he was anxious; Karen's model discounted such a pursuit. Kathy, Paul's client, indicated that she was helped by something quite foreign to Paul's structural explanation of what was therapeutic. Nancy, Mike's client, perceived Mike's attempt at demonstrating respect as a sign of immaturity. Mike's orientation did not account for the different ways that clients might interpret *his* behavior.

These early contradictions rarely pose a serious challenge to one's chosen model of treatment. Having struggled to select a guiding model, therapists are reluctant to let go of its assumptions. The validity assigned to the given approach continues to take precedence over the therapist's experience, and the client's idiosyncracies. Therapeutic outcome, after all, is generally reliable with any chosen model: Some get better, some drop out or get worse, and others stay the same.

The clients who get better tend to be those who are compliant to the extent that they can accommodate themselves to the therapist's model of psychotherapy. The accommodation process goes something like this: (1) The client presents with a complaint and possibly some specific notions about what may be causing the problem; (2) The therapist listens to the presenting complaint and reformulates the cause of the complaint (and possibly the complaint itself) into terms that are consistent with the therapist's guiding model. Within the framework of the therapist's model, the causes of the complaint are identified; whether or not the hypothesized causes are shared is a decision dictated by the therapist's orientation. A treatment plan is proposed and sometimes agreed upon. (4) The activities or behaviors that the therapist incorporates in treatment are determined by the formal theory that explains and predicts client responses.

Despite the security of the approach and the general predictability of outcome, clinical contradictions persist. In time, it becomes painfully evident that the selected model has limitations—often major—that do not reasonably explain the range of cases that a clinician typically encounters. Caseloads routinely include clients that should get better, according to the model, but don't (Karen and Jim), clients who get better for reasons the model doesn't explain (Paul and Kathy), and clients who respond to methods that the model doesn't accommodate (Mike and Nancy). Grappling with pragmatic evidence that contradicts theory, illusions are allowed to fade away, and the inherent complexity of clinical practice is truly recognized. Left with a more seasoned perspective, values, priorities, and frames of reference are reexamined and challenged. The search is renewed for a reliable but flexible intellectual framework to guide the therapeutic process.

This book is written for the therapist struggling to integrate clinical experience and the diversity of available techniques into a coherent framework for intervention. Coming from different disciplines (social work, psychology) and initially trained in various orientations (structural, behavioral, neoanalytical, and strategic), we found common ground in the developmental process described earlier. Early on, we each succumbed to the tendency to focus on those cases that appeared to confirm the reliability of our chosen models.

"Failures" were too often attributed to client variables such as "resistance," "poor motivation," "psychological unsophistication," or the host of other reasons therapists have been known to offer to justify poor outcome or general client unwillingness to continue in therapy for much more than four to seven sessions. Less often, we blamed ourselves, citing our inexperience, incompetency, learning deficits, and training deficiencies. Despite our heroic efforts to protect the sanctity of our chosen model(s), continued "failures" forced recognition of the inadequacies of our theoretical descriptions and the limitations of our expertise.

Our clients provided us with opportunities to reassess our work and served as powerful influences to search for more satisfactory and effective descriptions in the literature. Clients like Jim, Kathy, and Nancy taught us that theoretical models have limited applicability, that the therapeutic relationship is often more valued than our expert interventions, and that what our clients think and feel is far more relevant than our favored academic conceptualizations. This book attempts a pragmatic application of these simple, but difficult experiential lessons to the practice of individual, couple, and family therapy.

In writing this book, we have tried to avoid three pitfalls that characterize many books in this field. The first is the presentation of clinical anecdotes with little discussion of the rationale for intervention or the therapeutic process itself. These "cookbooks" often seem to be describing magic and rarely relate the work to the rest of the literature. The next pitfall is the book that elaborates an intricate theory base, describes the therapeutic process with tremendous insight, and extensively cites the literature, but fails to *translate* the theory, insight, and literature base to a specific or pragmatic level that enables replication. These books are difficult to plod through and leave the reader questioning what the authors really do when the office doors are closed. The final pitfall is the individual psychotherapy book or family therapy book that is written as if the other literature base is virtually nonexistent, thereby limiting the opportunity for useful cross-pollinization. We have strived to avoid these pitfalls by striking a balance between "academic" and clinical perspectives, and providing many crossover points between the individual and systemic literatures, including the illustration of our approach with individual, couple, and family case examples.

Preparing this book has been a challenging task. In addition to our clients, many people have contributed to this volume in many different ways. Student and trainee questions have enabled us to clarify what we do, colleagues' critiques permitted us to address the limitations of our approach, and many authors whose ideas have influenced our own (especially John Weakland, Paul Watzlawick, Jay Haley, C. H. Patterson, Steve de Shazer, Harry Goolishian, Carl Rogers, Barbara Held, and their colleagues) provided us with the inspiration to continue thinking about what we are doing messing around in people's lives. We are grateful to Carole Lang, Debrah Stafford, Kimberly Kremer, John Wolbert, Jay Slayden, and Peggy Volters, students in the marital and family program at Wright State University, for their persistent enthusiasm for ideas. We are especially grateful to Shelley Lopez and Sharon Trekell for their helpful suggestions on the manuscript. We owe a great debt to our colleagues and friends, Joseph Rock and Gregory Bernhardt, for critiquing the manuscript and strengthening its message. Also, thanks go to Steve Drewry for his skillful editorial help and to John Murphy, Paul Bruening, Mark Hubble, Brent Lawyer, Bernadine Parks, and Linda Heinz for their comments, suggestions, and support. Two people deserve special mention. Dottie Moynihan contributed to this project in a variety of ways. She tirelessly read draft after draft, compiled the appendices, figures, and tables, participated in many discussions, and generally helped clear the cobwebs during difficult times. Deserving our deepest appreciation is the office manager of the Dayton Institute for Family Therapy, Alice Penney, whose friendship, stability, and competence has provided a source of strength for many years. Finally, to our families, to whom this book is dedicated, thank you for your (almost) unending patience./lt/

Contents

CHANGING THE RULES

A CLIENT-DIRECTED APPROACH
TO THERAPY

1   Introduction: Empirical Influences

OUR common struggle with therapeutic failures provided the impetus for an ongoing search of the literature for more satisfying descriptions of clinical practice. An exploration of the literature encouraged new ways of thinking and acting, validated our clinical experiences, and initiated an evolving set of values and therapeutic actions concerning the therapeutic relationship. We have been heavily influenced by three seemingly disparate sources. Eclecticism, common factors, and brief therapy provide an empirical context for the evolution of our thinking and a rationale for the approach that we propose.

ECLECTICISM

A historical review of the psychotherapy literature leads to the disappointing recognition that any given model that purports to explain, predict, and ameliorate human suffering is limited in its applicability. Early on, the response to the problem of inadequate models was the development of rival schools of psychotherapy, characterized by a theoretical content specific to that particular point of view. Thus, over the course of the past 70 years, psychotherapists have not suffered a dearth of models from which to order the therapeutic process; by one recent count (Corsini, 1981), over 250 distinct systems of psychotherapy have been identified. While the disparities in approach are legion, all share one common feature: limited applicability. The up side, of course, is that under certain circumstances a given approach may be highly efficacious. The lure of increasing the efficacy, applicability, and efficiency of psychotherapy through the selective application of disparate techniques and models has fueled interest in the development of eclectic, or integrative, strategies for practice.

While eclectic practice dates to the first half of the century (Patterson, 1989), it is only in the past 20 years that eclecticism has been identified as a clearly delineated area of interest (Norcross, 1986). A variety of studies report that one-third to one-half of present-day clinicians prefer to label themselves as eclectic, disavowing affiliation with any particular therapeutic school (Garfield & Kurtz, 1977).

Although the term *eclecticism* lacks a singular precise definition and has, thus, been inconsistently and indiscriminantly applied, it does appear to retain several identifiable connotations: a stated dislike for a single orientation, selection from two or more theories, and the belief that present theoretical formulations are inadequate to explain or predict all observable behaviors (Garfield & Kurtz, 1977). These connotations were not only congruent with our clinical experiences, but also encouraged the pursuit of a flexible methodology for practice that could combine the best of what the individual psychotherapy and family therapy literature has to offer.

Eclecticism versus Integration versus Common Factors

Three main thrusts are evident in the modern movement to combine psychotherapy approaches (Saltzman & Norcross, 1990). Eclecticism in psychotherapy usually refers to the technical, largely atheoretical combination of clinical methods (Norcross, 1991). Technical eclecticism is empirical in the pragmatic selection of existing strategies on the basis of demonstrated efficacy. Technical eclecticism, therefore, endorses the use of a variety of techniques within a preferred theory base, without the necessity of a connection between metabeliefs and technique (Lazarus, 1967). A combination of approaches occurs at the level of specific procedure rather than at the level of theory. As exemplified by Lazarus (1981) and Beutler (1983), technical eclecticism strives to select the most useful procedures from the plethora of those available, irrespective of the theoretical underpinnings.

Another thrust, *integration*, denotes those efforts that seek the conceptual synthesis of varied psychotherapy theories (Saltzman & Norcross, 1990). The focus is more theoretical than empirical, and the emphasis is on the development of superordinate or metatheoretical models of psychotherapy. Integration addresses the distance between approaches by building a bridge that unites them (Norcross, 1991). As exemplified by Prochaska and DiClemente (1984) and Wachtel (1977), integration reconceptualizes and recombines aspects of different approaches into a new structure, at a higher order of synthesis, which shares some similarities to each approach, but possesses its own logic and coherence (Norcross, 1991).

Despite the emphasis on the differences among approaches, which at times overshadow and obscure commonalities, a number of writers recognize the significance of those elements common to diverse approaches. *Common-factor approaches*, the third thrust, seek to determine the core ingredients across therapies with the goal of constructing more efficacious treatments based upon these commonalities (Frank, 1973, 1982; Garfield, 1986; Patterson, 1989). Common-factor approaches strive to identify and operationalize those aspects of psychotherapy process that characterize successful approaches as a foundation for any treatment model.

The Thrust of This Book

This book presents an approach that incorporates aspects of all three thrusts to combine psychotherapy models. This approach seeks to (1) direct the selective application of diverse techniques irrespective of their theoretical underpinnings; (2) promote an integration of different theories through the *client's* idiosyncratic synthesis of various views introduced by the therapist; and (3) operationalize those factors that cut across theories and account for successful outcome. Because we combine components from all three thrusts, without regard to their theoretical compatibility, we will hereafter refer to our approach as an eclecticism.

While the intellectual appeal of theoretical integration is compelling, fundamental philosophical and conceptual incompatibilities constitute a formidable obstacle to the development of a unified, integrated system of psychotherapy (Goldfried & Newman, 1986). The content differences among approaches may suggest that technical eclecticism may provide the least obstructed route to the flexible application of diverse methods. In many ways, efforts at theoretical integration, or the search for a unified system of psychotherapy, is reminiscent of our earlier pursuits of an inherently right way to practice. Technical eclecticism, however, does not fully characterize our approach because conceptualizations derived from different theories, as well as specific techniques, are also included in the treatment process on the basis of their situational applicability. Consequently, an integration or synthesis of disparate theories can be said to occur, but it occurs from the frame of reference of the client, rather than from that of the therapist.

Restating the thrust of integration (see earlier) from the vantage point of the client: Clients reconceptualize problem experiences by combining aspects of their experience with alternative views introduced in therapy, creating new meaning structures, and containing their own logic to possibly allow for problem resolution. Integration from this perspective is an idiosyncratic, process-determined synthesis of ideas formulated by the client, essentially a new theory that emerges with explanatory and predictive validity for the client's specific circumstance.

While it embraces the philosophy and flexibility of technical eclecticism and promotes integration of theory from the vantage point of the client, the core element and primary emphasis of the approach of this book is the operationalization of the so-called common factors and the enhancement of other factors demonstrated of significance to successful outcome. The common factors literature presents a strong case for the assertion that the much sought after bridge among theories of psychotherapy may already indeed exist.

COMMON FACTORS

Patterson (1989) suggests that while most attempts at eclecticism focus on the inclusion of disparate methods and techniques, those factors that are common among therapies may provide a more useful foundation for an eclectic model. He makes a convincing argument that a systematic eclecticism must be based on those specific factors, common to all major theories, that have been supported by an ongoing and extensive body of research. Lending support to Patterson's argument, Goldfried and Safran (1986) similarly suggest that the integration of diverse approaches may be most fruitful when attempted at the "intermediate" level of abstraction, that is, the level at which common principles of change operate. Likewise, Garfield (1986) calls for an eclecticism based in the common factors that characterize successful approaches to psychotherapy.

Supportive of these arguments is the outcome literature, much of which suggests that positive outcome is, in large part, related to "common factors" (empathy, warmth, acceptance, encouragement, etc.) rather than specific technique. Lambert's (1986) review identifies that as much as 30% of outcome variance is related to these common elements. This figure is consistent with the 25–40% figures that Patterson (1984) cites. Lambert goes on to indicate that orientation-specific factors (technique) have been found to be no more powerful than placebo effect, both of which account for approximately 15% of positive outcome variance. Accounting for the remaining 40% of the variance are what Lambert identifies as spontaneous remission variables such as out of therapy events, client ego strength, and other client-specific variables. This research certainly challenges the propensity to hold onto the inherent and invariant validity of a chosen model, especially because orientation/technique are only as significant as placebo. Even more disconcerting is the implication that our specific orientations are largely insignificant when compared to common factors and client variables.

Patterson (1959) suggests a classification system that permits closer examination of the potency of the so-called common or nonspecific factors. Variables such as the therapist's authority, status, expertise, attractiveness, and credibility, as well as techniques such as persuasion, suggestion, encouragement, reassurance, and guidance are truly nonspecific and effectively constitute the placebo variables. While placebo has traditionally been ignored as a potent variable, Lambert's (1986) work suggests that placebo is at least as powerful a variable in positive outcome as is specific technique. Attempting to enhance placebo by design may as much as double the effectiveness of any intervention strategy. Recognizing and attending to client expectations and demand characteristics may secure, in part, the therapeutic alliance necessary for psychotherapy to proceed.

The second cluster of variables that Patterson identifies includes factors such as therapist acceptance, permissiveness, warmth, respect, nonjudgmentalism, honesty, genuineness, and empathic understanding. Patterson (1989) argues that these factors, which may be summarized as empathic understanding, respect, and therapeutic genuineness, are both specific and potent, providing at least the necessary basis for a facilitative interpersonal relationship. While disagreement exists regarding the extent to which these factors are sufficient for positive outcome, little disagreement exists among psychotherapists as to the importance and necessity of these qualities to the therapeutic process. Recognition of the importance of these specific therapist variables to positive outcome undercuts the view that expertise in methods and techniques is the critical factor in achieving client change. Rather, this body of evidence suggests that the therapist's influence lies in providing the conditions under which the client engages in behavioral or attitudinal change (Patterson, 1989).

Operationalizing Common Factors

Given the robust nature of the outcome results related to common therapist factors, as well as the nonspecific placebo variables, it would seem that any other elements incorporated into a systematic eclecticism should be consistent with and attempt to enhance those factors. Consistency with these factors would require that interventions be directed by the internal frame of reference of the client, rather than imposed by the therapist's theoretical frame of reference.

Understanding the client's subjective experience and phenomenological representation of the presenting complaint, and placing that experience above the theoretical predilection of the therapist, is a concept that appears to be consistent with the notion of enhancing common factors, both specific and nonspecific. The idea of operationalizing these factors provided a major thrust in the evolution of our thinking. The primacy of the client's experience and reality is the central organizing element of our work.

This book will propose a methodology for operationalizing common factors so that their effects may be enhanced and positive outcome encouraged. The proposal will (1) expand the definitions of empathy, respect, and genuineness to enable therapist actions beyond stereotypical responses; (2) articulate the process of accepting the client's frame of reference as the therapist's theoretical orientation; (3) introduce a therapist behavior called "validation," which explicitly seeks to high-light, legitimize, and "validate" the client's subjective experience; and (4) challenge the distinction between relationship and technique by extending the common factors context of the therapeutic relationship to the client's social environment through the intervention process itself. This book will also present a perspective that not only recognizes and empowers spontaneous remission effects, but also attempts to create opportunities for such effects to occur.

BRIEF PSYCHOTHERAPY

During the past ten years, there has been a growing interest in time-limited or brief approaches to psychotherapy. While traditional models may favor long-term treatment as an ideal model, reviews of client expectations, (Garfield, 1971) and treatment duration (Garfield, 1971, 1978; Koss, 1979; Langsley, 1978; Matarazzo, 1965) suggest that in actuality, practice is time-limited rather than long-term. By and large, the literature indicates that most outpatient therapy is limited to fewer than ten sessions per case; Budman and Gurman (1988) argue that this has been the case for several decades, citing Rubenstein and Lorr's (1956) findings in that regard.

While long-term therapy may represent the ideal of many clinicians, therapists have been remarkably unsuccessful at convincing clients to commit to long-term psychotherapy. Recent changes in the health care delivery and insurance systems has increased the pressure on therapists and consumers alike to establish a treatment focus that expedites the resolution of psychological and familial problems and contains the costs associated with such treatment. Caps on outpatient mental health care benefits, cuts in government funding, and managed mental health care plans will continue to push for treatment options that are not only therapeutically effective but also cost-effective. Like it or not, therapist behaviors are being affected by the pressures of the larger systems within which they operate.

Brief Therapy and Outcome Research

There is a growing body of evidence that appears to support the effectiveness of psychotherapy in general, and brief approaches (whether planned or unplanned) in particular. Given that the majority of outcome research has involved therapy that has lasted for short periods by the standards of traditional psychotherapy, virtually every major review of the efficacy of various individual therapies (e.g., Bergin, 1971; Bergin & Lambert, 1978; Lambert, Shapiro, & Bergin, 1986; Luborsky, Chandler, Auerbach, Cohen, & Bachrach, 1971; Orlinsky & Howard, 1986) has been an unacknowledged review of unplanned brief therapy (Budman & Gurman, 1988). These studies offer impressive evidence supporting the general effectiveness of unplanned brief individual psychotherapy. Similarly, the research literature on the effectiveness of marital and family therapy has shown comparable findings (Gurman & Kniskern, 1978; Gurman, Kniskern, & Pinsof, 1986).

Also supportive of brief therapy is the research suggesting a course of diminishing returns in psychotherapy with more and more effort required to achieve a noticeable difference in improvement (Orlinsky & Howard, 1986). Smith, Glass, and Miller (1980) similarly found the major impact of individual psychotherapy to occur in the first six to eight sessions, followed by a continuing, but decreasing, positive impact for the next ten sessions. In individual psychotherapy the largest proportion of positive change appears to occur in a time frame (six to eight sessions) that roughly parallels the amount of time most clients expect to stay in treatment (six to ten sessions; Garfield, 1971, 1978) and actually do stay in treatment (six to eight sessions; Garfield, 1978, 1986).

Compared to the enormous amount of research that exists on unplanned brief psychotherapy, outcome studies of planned brief therapy are few. The existing comparative studies of short-term versus long-term individual therapy show no reliable differences in effectiveness between the two (Butcher & Koss, 1978; Koss & Butcher, 1986; Luborsky, Singer, & Luborsky, 1975; Orlinsky & Howard, 1986). A parallel picture can be drawn from the existing studies of time-unlimited versus time-limited marital and family therapy (Gurman & Kniskern, 1978).

Brief Therapy versus Long-Term Therapy

The brief therapy literature addressing the comparable outcome of short-versus long-term therapy, the average length of treatment across treatment settings, client expectations concerning length of treatment, and the time frame in which the greatest proportion of change occurs is difficult to ignore. While the literature is convincing, and it is evident that our philosophy, values, and methods are aligned with those of brief therapy, the framework that follows in no way demands an either/or, brief-therapy/long-term therapy allegiance. The design is to empower common factor effects, enhance flexibility, and expand the repertoire of intervention strategies within a coherent framework for practice. It is our hope that regardless of one's position related to long- and short-term therapy, the approach may be of value to any clinician who seeks these same goals.

The book, however, presents an approach that is usually brief—not because of a fixed a priori number of sessions determined by the therapist—but rather because the acceptance of the client's frame of reference as the guiding theory for intervention necessarily shortens the treatment process most of the time. Brevity, therefore, is not advocated solely for the sake of being brief, but rather is a consequence of thinking and acting in a particular way with clients. This book asserts a therapeutic position that enables the rapid resolution of problems, but that respects the client's right to determine length of treatment.

EVALUATING THIS BOOK

Three sources of influence were discussed that have set an empirical context for the approach that follows. The three sources also provide a way for the reader to evaluate the approach of this book. The *eclecticism* literature highlights the explanatory and predictive inadequacy of any one theoretical school and emphasizes the advantages of combining multiple models of therapy. Given the noted difficulties with the achievement of an actual theoretical integration, a technical eclecticism, expanded by the selective use of conceptualizations from different theories as well as techniques, may offer the most direct route to the consideration of multiple options for intervention. Such an eclecticism may be significantly strengthened if it also includes those elements that cut across approaches that contribute to successful outcome.

The eclecticism literature also suggests criteria for evaluation of the approach that follows. Goldfried and Newman (1986) identify five themes that warrant consideration in any eclecticism or integration effort: (1) the potential complementarity of divergent approaches to therapy; (2) the interactive significance of cognition, behavior, and affect; (3) the need for a common theoretical language; (4) the elucidation of universal, metatheoretical principles of human change; and (5) the desire for empirically based procedure. As you read this book, evaluate whether or not the approach adequately addresses these recurrent themes of eclecticism.

The *common-factors* literature unequivocally supports the therapist variables of empathy, respect, and genuineness as a core foundation of any eclectic effort. Second only to client variables, these common factors account for much of positive outcome, and are far more important than technique. Empowering common factor effects through operationalizing therapist variables of empathy, respect, and genuineness beyond standby reflections and into the intervention process constitutes a core element of this approach.

Our assertions regarding the operationalization of common factors can be easily evaluated by keeping two questions in mind: (1) Does this approach specify therapist behaviors and values that demonstrate empathy, respect, and genuineness beyond stereotypical therapist responses? (2) Does this approach extend the common factors context of the therapeutic relationship into the intervention process itself?

The *brief psychotherapy* literature, especially the comparable outcome of short-term and long-term therapy and the mean number of sessions (ten) over the last three decades, provides a compelling argument for the clinician of any orientation to consider planning brief therapy rather than conducting brief therapy by default (Budman & Gurman, 1988). Brief therapy occurs as a frequent result of the therapist placing higher value on the client's frame of reference than any theoretical orientation; brief therapy emerges as a natural consequence from a rapid-change context set by the therapist's attitudes and behaviors regarding therapy, people, and the process of change.

The brief therapy literature also suggests criteria for evaluation of the approach in this book. Budman and Gurman (1988) summarize the value ideals of the brief therapist as: (1) the brief therapist begins treatment by using the least radical procedure, that is, therapy begins with the least costly, least complicated, and least invasive treatment; (2) the brief therapist views cure as inconceivable; (3) brief therapists view people as malleable and as constantly changing and developing; (4) the brief therapist, while maintaining an appreciation for the role of psychiatric diagnosis, has a health rather than an illness orientation; (5) the brief therapist takes the patient's presenting problem seriously and hopes to facilitate changes in some of the areas that the patient specifies or comes to clarify as important; (6) the brief therapist realizes that he or she may not be thanked for changes that have occurred after therapy, and may not, after relatively few visits, ever see the patient again; (7) the brief therapist assumes that psychotherapy may be "for better or for worse" and that not everyone who requests treatment needs or can benefit from it; and (8) finally, and most important, being in the world is seen as far more important than being in therapy. As you experience this book, evaluate our approach in terms of its consistency with the value ideals.

The confluence of the three sources provided the impetus for the approach to eclecticism in the ensuing chapters. Chapter 2 lays the groundwork and proposes a "process constructive" theory base for our eclecticism. Chapter 3 will present three pragmatic assumptions derived from theoretical foundations discussed in Chapter 2. Chapter 4 addresses the all-important first interview. Chapters 5 and 6 present intervention strategies that operationalize common factors, as well as enable the informed use of diverse theories and methods. Chapters 7 and 8 present full-length case studies. Ethical considerations and guidelines are presented in Chapter 9, as well as a gender perspective of our approach. Chapter 10 will provide our analysis of the three proposed evaluation methods and will conclude with our perspective on the future of psychotherapy.

2 ⬚ Theoretical Foundations

THE framework for eclectic practice presented in this book has evolved from the context described in Chapter 1 as well as earlier efforts to utilize and extend the strategic model of the Mental Research Institute (MRI) (Fisch, Weakland, & Segal, 1982; Watzlawick, Weakland, & Fisch, 1974) to include the contributions of other approaches. In the early 1980s, the senior author investigated the possibilities of integrating the MRI strategic approach with other models of family therapy. With the use of the construct of the homeostatic or protective function of symptoms as an example, an integration was suggested that permitted the selection of constructs from a variety of models of family therapy as metaphors to design strategic intervention (Duncan, 1984). The selective integration of concepts from outside the realm of strategic therapy served as the trigger for an evolutionary process of seeking a method of combining the best of what the psychotherapy literature has to offer.

Barbara Held (1984) was among the first to consider the advantages of combining an MRI approach with other models of psychotherapy. She proposed a "strategic eclecticism" and advocated the use of the MRI's resistance minimizing interventions to enhance compliance to therapeutic directives of other orientations.

Held's work was particularly helpful and influential to the senior author's work in a behaviorally oriented stress management program at a community mental health center. Held's strategic eclecticism provided a means to introduce strategic intervention into the stress management program and served as an impetus for a proposed integration between the MRI model and cognitive–behavioral approaches (Duncan, Rock, & Parks, 1987).

That early integration effort, which was referred to as "strategic-behavioral therapy," stressed the similarities between the two approaches.

We became enamored of the idea that similarities between models could provide a crossover point that allowed conceptual and practical integration of diverse approaches. Exploration of the literature of many disparate models invariably yielded many crossover points of concept and action between strategic therapy and the model under scrutiny. Although the notion of integration through similarities ran into roadblocks, looking for commonalities served to encourage an openness to ideas from the most antithetical of approaches.

Held (1986) expanded her proposal for a strategic eclecticism by suggesting that the MRI problem formation model is relatively void of specific theoretical content, thereby allowing the use of theoretical content from any approach in service of strategic goals. Held elaborated a process-content distinction that extended our earlier notion of selecting frames from other approaches as metaphors for intervention. Her distinction also enabled the recognition that the process-oriented strategic model could provide an organizing component for an eclectic approach that went beyond the confines of the strategic-behavioral pairing or the pairing of any two approaches (Duncan & Parks, 1988). The process-content distinction added both depth and support to the use of a constructivist rationale for selecting alternative meaning from various psychotherapy orientations.

In retrospect, a theme of simple flexibility emerged from a 10-year search for theoretical formulations that would expand the strategic model of MRI and permit an eclecticism. Constructivism provides a relative and contextual perspective of the therapeutic relationship that not only demystifies psychotherapy models as no more than views of reality that structure the therapist's reality, but, more important, also provides a strong rationale for the primacy of the client's view over the therapist's theoretical orientation. Buckley's (1967) description of sociocultural systems suggests a view of system interaction that emphasizes the flexibility of process and deemphasizes the rigidity and restrictions of a purely homeostatic perspective of system operation. The MRI problem formation model eliminates the encumbrances of pathology-based explanatory schemes of client dilemmas, allowing for a more idiosyncratic and client-specific formulation of both the presenting complaint and the client's goal for change. Finally, Held's process-content distinction enables the consideration of multiple theoretical contents without the limitations inherent in the invariant application of any one theory.

CONSTRUCTIVISM

The philosophical position of constructivism and social construction theory from psychology (Gergen, 1985) both suggest that reality develops phenomenologically, emerging from the constructs of the observer-describer and his or her interaction with the environment. Reality is therefore invented, not discovered (Watzlawick, 1984) and is evident only through the constructed meanings that shape and organize experience. People, as meaning-generating systems, create meaning through a flowing interaction of ideas and correlated actions. The generation of meaning is an interactive and highly idiosyncratic process that emerges from the subjective phenomenology of the individual. These constructed realities organize perception and experience into rule-governed patterns or meaning systems through which individuals may describe, direct, and predict their lives (Duncan, Parks, & Rusk, 1990).

Meaning is created in two ways (Buckley, 1967). Meaning is neither inherent solely in external experience nor the internal state of the individual, but rather is constructed during the ongoing interaction between the individual and the social environment. Varela (1989) describes this level of meaning creation as emerging as a result of effective action in the natural world.

The human capacities for symbol manipulation and self-awareness enable another avenue of meaning construction. People can experience a transaction entirely at a covert or internal level that permits the continuous generation of meaning apart from the interpersonal experience.

Accordingly, meaning systems may be generated through the transactional experience (the individual's interaction in the social environment), its covert rehearsal or internal processing, and the ordering and organizing of both ways. Through social interpretation and the intersubjective influence of language, family, and culture, an evolving set of meanings emerge unendingly from the interactions among people (Anderson & Goolishian, 1988).[1]

Thinking of reality as meanings created in dynamic social exchange and communicative interaction can be both mind-boggling and disconcerting at the same time. Much confusion has arisen from esoteric descriptions of constructivism and the application of an antirealist epistemology to psychotherapy. We would like to cut through the esoterica and reach the bottom line for eclectic practice.

Implications

Constructivism, not in the radical sense, but in the common sense variety applied to therapy, does not deny the existence of objects, events, or

---

[1]Regrettably, Harry Goolishian suddenly passed away on November 11, 1991. His driving intellectual curiosity and continual theoretical innovations will be sorely missed.

experiences, but rather provides a challenging commentary on the relative and context-bound nature of meanings ascribed to those objects, events, and experiences by an observer. Understood in this way, constructivism elevates the client's view of reality, particularly the client's meaning system regarding the presenting problem, to paramount importance in the therapeutic process. Applying constructivism to therapy allows the client's meaning system to transcend to a hierarchically superior position to the therapist's theoretical orientation and/or personal beliefs. Constructivism, therefore, provides a strong rationale for respecting the preeminence of the client's world view. It suggests that the therapeutic process is best served by meeting clients within their idiosyncratic meaning systems regarding their problem experiences (Solovey & Duncan, 1992).

From a constructivist vantage point, theoretical language and content conceptualizations may be viewed as somewhat arbitrary metaphorical representations that explain and organize the therapist's reality and may have little in common with the client's perception and interpretation of the presenting concern. The very content or theoretical orientation that the therapist selects to order the therapeutic reality necessarily limits the search for solutions. A constructivist position deemphasizes the importance of the search for undeniable truths as well as the role of the therapist as the source of such truths. Constructivism, therefore, encourages more flexibility in the therapist reality and consequently facilitates an eclectic framework of intervention.

Constructivism also provides a different language of how change occurs. The language of meaning systems enables a respectful and noninterfering vocabulary for change that permits the therapist role to be essentially collaborative, and instrumental only in the sense of creating the conditions for change, not the actual change itself. A meaning systems perspective deemphasizes therapist power, control, and a covertly directive or manipulative stance with clients. We will return to this implication of a constructivist stance in our discussion of pragmatic assumptions in Chapter 3, as well as in Chapter 9 in a discussion of ethics and strategic therapy.

PROCESS LEVEL SYSTEMS

Buckley, in a classic discussion (1967), categorized systems at three levels of description, each applicable to a specific domain. Buckley's scheme of systems is useful because it allows the consideration of different ways of thinking about systems based in the particular kind of system under concern.

It is Buckley's third level, the process/adaptive level (hereafter called *process*) that describes sociocultural systems such as families. At the social systems level, process or dynamic interaction between and among system members is primary. Structure is a fluid and ever-changing representation of an ongoing process, rather than a fixed, static entity. Structure is therefore no more than a snapshot of transactional process and continuously changing relationships. Unlike biological systems, which are characterized by fixed structures that perform recognizable and invariant functions across systems (e.g., the hypothalamus [structure] and temperature regulation [function]), social systems are possessed of no immediately identifiable fixed structures of invariant function (Buckley, 1967; Duncan & Fraser, 1987).

Inherent to process-level systems is the capacity for evolution and elaboration. These systems are not only sensitive to variation in the social environment but are also essentially dependent on change for continued viability. Unlike biological systems, which are characterized by mechanisms that reduce and eliminate variability, social systems rely on variation to stimulate interactional process, the construction of individual and shared meaning, as well as the continual movement toward complexity, flexibility, and differentiation. A sociocultural system, then, is a meaning-processing system of dynamic social exchange through which individuals accommodate or assimilate ongoing change (variation) in the internal and external social environment.

Implications

Buckley's process-level system represents a significant departure from the prevailing descriptions of family systems found in the literature. The majority of family therapy approaches are based in a biological level of system description and emphasize, to varying degrees, the concepts of structure, symptom function, and homeostasis. The process-level view provides a flexibility of thought and action that is not encumbered by a necessary and invariant search for homeostatic mechanisms and the like. Adopting a process view allows multiple courses of conceptualization and intervention that include consideration of homeostasis without the restriction of its sole reliance (Duncan, 1984; Fraser, 1984a, 1986). The process-level description of systems, therefore, provides a theory base that enables an eclectic approach.

The emphasis on the interactional process surrounding variation and its importance to meaning construction is particularly relevant to psychotherapy. In general, the therapeutic goal is to promote conditions that increase choice and enhance possibilities for revisions of those meanings and/or experiences that the client views as problematic. In service of that goal and through the use of the therapeutic conversation and the therapist's suggestions, variation is introduced to the system. Variation then stimulates interactional process and meaning construction, thereby encouraging client change and systemic growth.

While most of the systems literature can be argued to flow from a biological level of system description, the strategic approach of the MRI seems to align with the process-level description. It is particularly the MRI's interactional perspective of problem process that enables an eclecticism.

MENTAL RESEARCH INSTITUTE: A PROBLEM PROCESS MODEL

The strategic approach of the MRI is an outgrowth of the family systems movement and essentially evolved concurrently with many approaches to family therapy. At a time during which several independent groups were studying families containing a schizophrenic member, the Bateson project investigated the communication patterns in schizophrenic families. This research culminated in the double-bind theory of schizophrenia (Bateson, Jackson, Haley, & Weakland, 1956). Until the double-bind hypothesis, most other family-oriented descriptions of human behavior were mired in awkward transformations of psychodynamic theories. The double-bind theory, based in communicative interaction, had the powerful capacity to describe human dilemmas as interactional in nature, and freed the emerging field from the constraints of the language of pathology (Anderson & Goolishian, 1988). Subsequently, Haley and Weakland, original members of the Bateson group, became interested in the work of Milton Erickson. After several years of studying Erickson's innovative methods, both Haley and Weakland went on to integrate Erickson's ideas with communication theory and cybernetics, forming the basis for what is now known as strategic therapy.

Main Principles

Weakland, Fisch, Watzlawick, and Bodin (1974) delineate the main principles of their work as: (1) the approach is symptom oriented, in a broad sense; (2) problems that bring people to psychotherapists are situational difficulties between people—problems of interaction; (3) problems are primarily an outcome of everyday difficulties, usually involving adaptation to some life change, that have been mishandled by the parties involved; (4) problems develop usually by overemphasis or underemphasis on difficulties in living; (5) once a difficulty begins to be seen as a "problem," the continuation and exacerbation of the problem results from the creation of a positive feedback loop, most often centering on those very behaviors of the individuals in the family that are intended to resolve the difficulty; (6) long-standing problems or symptoms are not viewed as "chronicity," but the persistence of a repetitively poorly handled difficulty; (7) resolutions of problems require a substitution of behavior patterns so as to interrupt the vicious, positive feedback circles; (8) means to such an interruption often may appear illogical or paradoxical; (9) accepting what the client offers and reversing usual treatment in a pragmatic fashion is the major focus of therapy; and (10) conceptions and interventions are based on direct observation of *what* is going on in systems of human interaction, *how* they continue to maintain the problem, and *how* they may be altered most effectively and efficiently.

In brief, the MRI holds that problems develop from chance or transitional circumstances encountered by individuals and families evolving through the life cycle. It is when adjustment or adaptation to a variation is perceived as a difficulty that problems develop. The MRI simply and eloquently suggests two conditions as necessary for problem development: (1) the mishandling of the difficulty and (2) upon failure of the original solution attempt, the application of more of the same, resulting in a vicious cycle (Watzlawick et al., 1974). The inter-/intra-personal interaction that surrounds the difficulty, the process by which individual and shared meaning related to the difficulty is constructed, and the interplay of both are seen as significant to the problem process. Idiosyncratic interpretations and perceptions both influence and are influenced by the difficulty itself, creating a problem-oriented system (Goolishian & Anderson, 1987), or one in which interpersonal interactions and meaning construction are organized around the problem. While presenting complaints and concerns may be highly content-laden and idiosyncratic to the individual or the situation, the *problem* is defined in terms of the interactive process. Problems, then, occur as part of a vicious cycle of attempts to adjust or adapt to an internally or externally initiated variation. The variation, once perceived as a difficulty, becomes not only the original difficulty, but also all the meanings it has accumulated through the course of those interacting around it. Based on the individual and shared meanings about the problem or how to solve it, people will try variations on a theme of the same solution pattern over and over again. This usually occurs despite the best intentions of those involved and the fact that the solution attempts are recognized as not helping. The solution, in essence, becomes the problem (Watzlawick et al., 1974).

Implications

Given that the MRI emphasizes the process of interaction surrounding the problem, and in general views all behavior as explainable in terms of its place in a wider ongoing sequence of communicative transaction in a social system, a very different set of assumptions regarding problem etiology emerges. A major assumption is that regardless of basic origins or ties to historical or personality variables, problems persist only if they are maintained by ongoing current behavioral sequences between the client and others with whom he or she interacts. Because etiology resides in the interactive process, models of psychopathology, such as DSM- III-R, are viewed as no more than explanatory schemes that structure and organize behavior that appears irrational or self-defeating to an observer. The human experience of emotional and interpersonal difficulties is normalized in a model that requires no deficits of either character or family structure. This simple but elegant interactional view enables a contextual perspective of human behavior that depathologizes problems in living.

The significance of removing pathology explanations can hardly be overstated. All therapeutic intervention relies on the premises to which the helper subscribes. These premises structure the therapeutic intervention at every level. How the therapist interprets and conceptualizes the clinical situation influences not only the nature of the helping relationship, but also what data will require focus, who will be seen in treatment, what will be said, and how results will be evaluated. A process-based perspective, such as that of the MRI, shifts the focus from curing or correcting character traits or deficiencies to empowering clients to utilize their existing resources to resolve problems.

Although the MRI does not present its model in terms of compatibility with other theoretical orientations, Held (1986) has argued that the MRI approach can subsume other individual and interpersonal models and, therefore, may be utilized as a basis for eclectic practice. Her argument rests in an important distinction between content and process elements within and across models of psychotherapy.

PROCESS VERSUS CONTENT

Held (1986), building on the work of Prochaska and DiClemente (1982), defines *process* as the activities or behaviors the therapist engages in to promote change or develop coping solutions (i.e., methods, techniques, interventions, strategies). Process embodies one's theory of how change occurs (Held, 1991). *Content* is the object of the change involving the aspects of the client and his or her behavior that the therapist decides to focus his or her interventions on (Held, 1991). *Content* is identified and defined at both *formal* and *informal* theoretical levels (Held, 1991). *Formal theory* consists of either general notions regarding the cause of problems (e.g., symptoms are surface manifestations of intrapsychic conflict; symptoms are homeostatic mechanisms regulating a dysfunctional subsystem) or predetermined and specific explanatory schemes (e.g., fixated psychosexual development; triangulation), which must be addressed *across* cases to solve problems. Cause and effect are either specified or implied by way of the theoretical constructs of the formal theory. Those constructs provide the content, which become the invariant explanations of the problems that bring clients to therapy.

Models of Psychotherapy

While all models of psychotherapy are built on theoretical content, they vary in the degree to which content is emphasized and elaborated (Held, 1991). Despite the fact that variation exists in the extent to which the therapeutic process is ordered by a particular orientation's content, most therapies tend to fall to the content-oriented pole of the content–process continuum. The client or clients will present a complaint or set of complaints to the therapist, and the therapist will overtly or covertly reinterpret the complaints within the language of the therapist's formal theory or theoretical content. The therapist reformulation of the complaint into a specific preconceived theoretical content will enable treatment to proceed down a particular path flowing from the formal theory. Consider how a client complaint of panic attacks may be viewed in terms of many content-oriented models, and how the selected model suggests a particular content path to follow. A psychodynamic clinician may view the problem as a result of repressed ideas and/or wishes intruding into consciousness. The therapist may pursue information from the specific stage of psychosexual development deemed relevant and make interpretations to allow the client to integrate the unconscious material that is requiring the anxiety attacks as a defense.

A cognitive clinician may view the problem as a result of a set of irrational beliefs and/or cognitive distortions that the person has learned. The therapist may pursue the client's self statements regarding the panic attacks and the situations in which the attacks occur, as well as the underlying beliefs and distortions that the self statements represent. The therapist may attempt to replace self-defeating thoughts with self-enhancing ones.

A structural family therapist may view the panic attacks as serving a homeostatic function for the client's marriage, in that the marriage is protected from conflict because of the couple's focus on the attacks. The therapist may refocus the problem as between the client and spouse and address the trust and intimacy issues that underlie the panic attacks, thereby eliminating the need for the symptom as a homeostatic mechanism.

An MRI therapist may view the panic attacks as a vicious cycle of unsuccessful solution attempts that the client and others with whom he or she interacts have employed. The therapist may pursue an interruption of the problem-maintaining process. The MRI is distinguished from the psychodynamic, cognitive, and structural approaches by an attention to the process surrounding the panic attacks and how that process may be interrupted. No particular or invariant content path to problem formation or maintenance is posited by the MRI.

Accordingly, the MRI model falls to the process-oriented pole of the content-process continuum. The MRI problem process model is a general and inclusive view of problem formation and maintenance, and posits no particular theoretical "true maintainer" or "real cause" of the presenting problem other than redundant solutions. The MRI-oriented therapist focuses on the vicious cycle of unsuccessful solution attempts. Unlike most therapies, which rely heavily on formal theoretical content to structure their understanding of the problem, the MRI position holds that the interactive process itself *is* the problem. The only goal that an MRI model dictates is that of changing the interactive process that constitutes and maintains the problem; the sole focus of therapy is on the problem process. As such, the content focus of psychotherapy can emerge from the *informal theory* of the client.

Informal Theory

Informal theory, which is evident at the client complaint level, involves the specific notions held by clients about the causes of their particular complaints. Revealed through statements such as "I guess I've always had really low self-esteem," "I've never been able to trust anyone, it goes back to when I was a kid," "He doesn't *really* talk to me," as well as the elaboration of such statements, informal theory is highly idiosyncratic. At times, the match between the formal theory held by the therapist and the informal theory held by the client may seem serendipitously congruent (e.g., a client presenting to a cognitive therapist with a statement such as "Despite what everyone tells me, I just don't seem to like myself very well; I can't get past the feeling that there is something really wrong with me.") More often, the informal theory of the client will be overtly or covertly reinterpreted within the language of the therapist's formal theory before treatment proceeds (recall the example of panic attacks).

Implications

Held's general content/process delineation, coupled with her identification of the MRI as a process-based model, suggests an avenue for an eclectic approach that could utilize content as a vehicle for change. For a client to articulate a complaint requires that it be conceptualized in a content-rich meaning system (i.e., the informal theory); even the most general and nonspecific of client-presented goals must be ordered by the content of the client's idiosyncratic meaning system. Client focus must necessarily be content oriented and value-laden. In content-oriented approaches to psychotherapy, the formal theoretical reality of the therapist exists in a hierarchically superior position to the informal theory of the client. This formal theory necessarily structures problem definition as well as outcome criteria. The more content oriented the approach, the more content directed the goals become. The MRI change model shifts therapist focus from content-oriented goals (e.g., shifting coalitions, establishing a rational belief system, correcting learning deficits, etc.) to process-based goals and outcome criteria. Given that the sole goal dictated by the MRI model is that of changing the problem-maintaining interactive process, the content-structured goals associated with the client's informal theory may be actively utilized in service of the process-oriented goals of the therapist. Techniques, methods, and intervention strategies may be selected from any of the available models that, at the content level, are congruent with the informal theory of the client.

THEORETICAL ASSUMPTIONS, PSYCHOTHERAPY, AND SHAVING LEGS?

The combination of a process perspective of systems, a constructivist view of reality and meaning generation, an interactional model of problem formation, and the distinction between process and content approaches serves as a basis for an eclecticism that accepts the informal theory of the client as hierarchically superior to the formal theory of the therapist. This process-oriented approach, when considered in the context of the inherent values associated with common factors, brief therapy, and eclecticism, suggests several assumptions regarding people, problems, and the practice of psychotherapy.

Consider your own set of assumptions as you read the following example and think about what intervention options unfold based upon your assumptions. In the first interview with a 20-year-old man, he describes a feeling in his face that is directed by the curvature of his spine, which either curves to God or to the devil. He also notes that his hands are not there at times, and that one of his legs is a woman's and one a man's.

From just that opening statement, many assumptions may quickly emerge regarding what the problem is and how it may best be treated. Many professionals may interpret the client's statement as an indication of a mental illness. Such a view would conceptualize the statement as a somatic delusion that probably results from some psychotic process in the individual. A biochemical imbalance involving the neurotransmitter dopamine would be hypothesized as the underlying mechanism of the behavior expressed in the session. This perspective may therefore suggest medical treatment (i.e., psychotropics, hospitalization, ECT, psychosurgery) perhaps combined with some form of psychosocial treatment to assist the individual and his family in managing the illness.

A more psychological view may conceptualize the client's presentation as a fundamental deficit in the individual's ability to form relationships such that the client's behavior reflects a return to early childhood forms of communication. His fragile ego, unable to handle the extreme stress of interpersonal challenges, has regressed. From this view, therapy would require the client to learn adult forms of communication and achieve insight into the role that the past has played. This process would occur very gradually, probably over a period of years.

A family systems view may conceptualize the client presentation as a reflection of dysfunction elsewhere in the client's family and as a homeostatic mechanism that detours conflict away from his parents' relationship. It is hypothesized that the young man may be protecting his parents and sacrificing his own development in the service of detouring their conflict. From this view, family therapy would address the conflict between the parents, restructure the cross-generational coalition, and attempt to eliminate the need for the client to protect his parents through the symptom.

Obviously, such differences in conceptualization and treatment of the proposed clinical situation also make for some radical differences in prognosis as well as in ramifications for the client and his family. The formal theory of the therapist not only dictates what sort of therapy is selected, but also how drastic and lengthy it is expected to be. Furthermore, the evaluation of outcome will also depend on the therapist's original construction of the client's presentation. If that original construction or formal theory says "schizophrenia," and the problem is viewed as an inherent and fundamental defect or disease process, the client may be forever labeled a schizophrenic, even if the peculiar behavior ceases that led to the initial construction (i.e., in remission). From another point of view, however, a change may be interpreted as an indication that the problem no longer exists.

There are literally 100 ways of conceptualizing the brief information given earlier, and the formal theories described, although presented in a grossly oversimplified fashion, have merit and warrant consideration. While they deserve consideration across cases, they do not merit invariant application across cases. The therapist who actually saw this client held a different set of assumptions about people, problems, and psychotherapy.

The therapist's process systemic view of the client's statement enables the therapeutic system (client and therapist) to be viewed as an ongoing exchange of meaning that continually shifts and changes as new information (variability) is added. The client statement was merely a snapshot of an ongoing transactional sequence that itself was in the process of change. The interaction between the therapist and client creates a context for meaning construction, and meaning may be cogenerated via the dynamic communicative exchange called psychotherapy.

The therapist's constructivist perspective suggests that the client had generated a meaning system that included a belief that God and the devil were within him and that he possessed characteristics of both males and females. The therapist accepted the statement at face value, believing that this client deserved no less acceptance and validation than any other client sharing concerns. The therapist placed the client's idiosyncratic meaning system above his own theoretical formulations.

The therapist's problem process assumption (from the MRI) viewed the ongoing interaction between the therapist and the client as significant to the client's expression of his dilemma. Although no one from the client's family was present, the therapist wondered *how* others have responded to the client and *what* solutions they have attempted to help him. A problem process perspective interpreted the client's presentation as a response to some developmental transition or incidental difficulty that the client's and other's efforts at solving were probably exacerbating.

The process-content distinction allowed the therapist to utilize the client's informal theory (the client description of the complaint) as a content-oriented frame of reference for intervention. The informal theory took precedence over any formal theory notions the therapist was contemplating.

In response to the client's presentation, the therapist asked the client which leg was the woman's leg. After the client indicated it was his left leg, the therapist asked him if he had shaved his woman's leg yet. The client got a quizzical look on his face, blushed, and then laughed. He said that he wasn't going to shave his damn leg. The session proceeded to a conversation about the client's struggles in leaving home, which included a major confrontation with his parents and minister and living in an abandoned car for the past week. The young man did not make another "delusional" comment the rest of the session.

The therapist's formal theory creates a powerful context within which psychotherapy unfolds. We are arguing for a formal theory that provides maximum flexibility and that discounts the invariant application of any particular therapeutic reality. In the case example, we are not denying the possibility of brain dysfunction or biochemical imbalance. On the contrary, this particular client did in fact take an antipsychotic for a

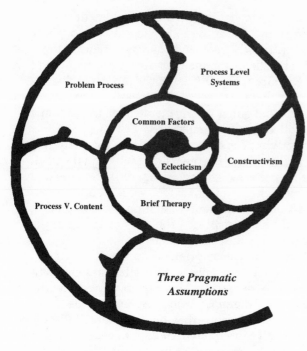

Eclecticism
- All models inadequately describe human experience
- All models have limitations in application

Common Factors
- Second only to client factors, accounts for much of positive outcome, far more than technique

Brief Therapy
- Comparable outcome with long-term therapy
- Average length of treatment across settings
- Client expectations of length of treatment
- When greatest proportion of change occurs

Constructivism
- Client's view (not therapist's) is primary to therapeutic process
- Theory is only a representation of reality, not a reflection of it
- Meaning evolves from social interaction and its rehearsal and recollection

Process Level Systems
- Process is primary
- Change is continuous
- Variation stimulates change

Problem Process
- Problems arise from interactional process, not pathology
- The solution is the problem

Process V. Content
- No true maintainers or real causes of human problems
- Informal theory dictates therapeutic content

FIGURE 2.1. Interacting empirical and theoretical segments evolving to form three pragmatic assumptions to guide clinical practice.

few months. Instead, we are suggesting that sole reliance on a biochemical view or any other theory severely limits intervention options and may preclude the therapist–client collaboration required for the co-construction of more helpful meanings.

In summary, this chapter has presented the formal theory of our proposed eclecticism: (1) Constructivism and Social Construction Theory; (2) Buckley's process level system description; (3) The MRI's problem process model; and (4) Held's process-content distinction. As illustrated in Figure 2.1, the empirical influences described in Chapter 1 and the theoretical foundation discussed in Chapter 2, form the segments that flow to the pragmatic assumptions of our approach. Chapter 3 will set the stage for the clinical application to follow through a practical discussion of these assumptions.

3 ▨ Pragmatic Assumptions

THREE pragmatic assumptions provide a practical and concrete interpretation of the theory for clinical practice. Chapter 3 explains *what* the theory means and *how* it is relevant when facing clients in distress, and also addresses the complex issue of how change occurs in psychotherapy. The assumptions are:

1. Problems, and their solutions, are embedded in the interactive process.
2. The client's presentation, rather than the therapist's orientation, determines therapy goals, the content of the therapeutic conversation, and intervention strategies.
3. Intervention interrupts the problem cycle, provides meaning revision opportunities, and validates the client's experience.

To facilitate the goal of explaining what the theory means and how it is relevant to clinical practice, two case examples are presented and used to illustrate each assumption. Additional vignettes also punctuate the major points.

CASE ONE[1]

Lynn, a 43-year-old woman, presented with concerns regarding her 9-year-old daughter's (Amy) irritability and unhappiness, which Lynn viewed as possible signs of a genetically transmitted depression. Lynn cited her own history of depression, as well as her mother's depression history, as evidence for an inherited, genetic depression in her daughter.

[1]Appendix B provides a quick reference to case illustrations and page numbers.

She stated that her efforts to comfort, reassure, and cheer the child were ineffective. She feared that these early signs would worsen, dooming Amy to the bouts of depression that had characterized the lives of the two previous generations. Given the strength of the client's beliefs regarding the biological, genetic risk to her daughter, as well as the client's implicit values regarding a mother's role, the therapist chose to intervene within the parameters of the client's meaning system, and accepted the client's view of depression. Accordingly, the therapist utilized clinical content derived from the literature on biological/genetic depression, and linked it to a diathesis-stress paradigm (Davison & Neale, 1986). The therapist suggested that, given the familial predisposition to depression, environmental factors could be critical in the expression of the predisposition. Because the depressive tendency appeared to be a given, perhaps the mother could assist her child in learning how to cope with her depression by encouraging the child's expression of her complaints, validating those complaints, and perhaps even exaggerating them somewhat. This would implicitly encourage the child to "work through" her feelings and develop competence in coping.

CASE TWO

Anita, a 26-year-old woman, entered therapy following a 2-week hospitalization for a suicide attempt. A diagnosis of Borderline Personality Disorder (BPD), of which Anita was aware, accompanied her, along with a detailed psychological evaluation recommending intensive long-term psychotherapy. Anita wanted to pursue an understanding of BPD and its historical origins in her childhood. The therapist respected the client's goals and discussed the client's experience of her childhood. After a few sessions, Anita began discussing areas of her life that were dissatisfying. She and the therapist explored her relationship with her husband and her feelings related to his lack of support, as well as her lack of fulfillment in her role as a housewife. At many junctures, Anita sadly commented on her desire to be different and her belief that her disorder would prevent any changes. Responding to the client's belief in the validity of diagnosis, as well as her strong desire to change, the therapist suggested that BPD was certainly one way of describing the sequence of events that led to the suicide attempt and that there were several other ways as well. The therapist then asked the client what if the diagnosis of BPD were incorrect—what would that mean? Anita responded that she would confront her husband, get a part-time job, and take a class at a local university.

1. PROBLEMS, AND THEIR SOLUTIONS, ARE EMBEDDED IN THE INTERACTIVE PROCESS

This assumption incorporates two aspects of "interactive process," the first being the interactive process surrounding the client's presenting concern and the second the interpersonal event of the therapist–client relationship.

Interactive Process: The Presenting Concern

Despite their relationship to the past or to personality or biological factors, all client concerns are continually being maintained and shaped by ongoing interaction in the social system (Watzlawick et al., 1974). Client concerns are part of a problem process characterized by the client's attempts to solve the concern, as well as the attempts of others to ameliorate the concern. The presenting complaint occurs in a context of interacting participants who maintain or change their views of themselves and their relationships through communicative interaction. Client concerns, then, represent contextually relevant meaning systems that are interactively generated via dynamic social exchange—both outside and inside of therapy.

Clients are evolving biopsychosocial entities who will inevitably encounter chance or transitional/developmental difficulties as they move through the individual, marital, and family life cycle. Problems arise from the interaction of the developing individual/family and the meanings ascribed to those random and transitional difficulties. They are maintained and exacerbated by vicious cycles of attempts to adjust to the difficulties. Whatever their origins, the problems that bring people to therapy are amenable to change through intervention in the ongoing interactional process (Watzlawick et al., 1974). Therapy, therefore, focuses on the behavioral and communicative interaction among participants in the problem system and between the meaning-creating individual and the environment.

Lynn

In the case of Lynn (Case One), the problem was viewed as embedded in the interactive process. The problem behaviors that Lynn was assigning the meaning of genetic depression were described as a general negative attitude, complaining, boredom, and sadness when unable to find a friend with whom to play. Lynn's solution attempts largely involved long discussions and lectures in which Lynn would attempt to comfort Amy and talk her out of her negativism. Lynn also went to great lengths to help her daughter not to be bored or sad. For example, Lynn at times called her daughter's friends to invite them over; she invented games to play; and in general, she spent much of her time monitoring the "depression" and trying to help her daughter overcome it. Sometimes Lynn took Amy shopping when she appeared sad. Lynn's persistent attempts to help her daughter perpetuated and exacerbated the very problem she was attempting to solve.

Also relevant was the meaning of genetic depression that Lynn generated to organize her experience of Amy's troubling behaviors. The constructed meaning of "genetic depression" limited Lynn's possible solution alternatives. The therapist focused on the interaction among participants in the problem process (Lynn's solution attempts of comforting, cheering, and lecturing), and the interaction between the meaning creating individual and the environment (i.e., Lynn's meaning system of genetic depression). The problem, therefore, was the behavioral interaction surrounding the daughter's unwanted behaviors, as well as the generated meaning that had emerged regarding the depression.

Anita

In the case of Anita (Case Two), the interactive process included all the participants' attempts to help Anita after her suicide attempt. This included her subsequent hospitalization and diagnosis of BPD, and the hospital therapist's recommendation that she and her husband consider her disorder in any decisions they may make. The therapist cautioned the husband against escalating arguments and advised him to remain calm always. The husband quickly accepted the diagnosis and the expert's advice and began fitting all of his wife's behavior into the framework of BPD. He removed many of Anita's responsibilities and treated her as if she were indeed fragile and incompetent, which, not surprisingly, infuriated Anita. Their interaction went something like this: Anita would raise a concern about her husband's family of origin or his tight grip on the checkbook. Anita's husband would remain calm at all costs and would repeat to Anita that she should calm down and relax, reminding her of her emotional disorder. Anita then would scream or throw things, her husband would become completely silent, and Anita would blame herself because of her BPD. Her husband always agreed.

Anita's interaction with others attempting to help her led to an emergent meaning that organized Anita's experiences and perceptions about her suicide attempt. That emergent meaning, namely the diagnosis of BPD, continued to influence and shape her interaction with her social environment and vice versa. The problem, therefore, was the behavioral interaction surrounding Anita's suicide attempt and subsequent hospitalization, and the generated meaning that was constructed about that attempt.

Pathology and Diagnosis

Because we are advocating a therapy that focuses on interactional process, individual or systemic pathology is not emphasized (although not ignored), nor are symptoms seen as *necessarily* functional to the individual or interpersonal system (Duncan, 1984). This is a nonpejorative and nonjudgmental view of people and problems. Attributions of pathology are viewed as generally unhelpful and potentially harmful. While ascriptions of functionality may be utilized (e.g., ascribing a protective function to a symptom), investment in the concept of functionality may limit therapeutic options. In a similar vein, diagnostic labels that construct the situation as either unchangeable or bearing a poor prognosis are avoided. This is not to say that the information that a diagnosis may yield should be ignored, but rather that such information may not be necessarily helpful and should be used discriminantly, based upon the idiosyncracies of the case under concern.

It is our value position that people *deserve* to be generally viewed as possessing the necessary resources and skills for problem improvement to occur unless overwhelming evidence to the contrary is presented. At the very least, a nonpejorative and nonjudgmental perspective encourages the creation of a change-enhancing therapeutic context, given the therapist's constructed meaning that change will occur. Such a position may also implicitly empower common factors because of the therapist's conveyed respect for the client's dignity as a competent individual inevitably capable of growth.

Pitfalls of Pathology

The impact of pathological labels can hardly be overestimated because of the potential disrespect they may represent and the dangers of chronicity and rigidity that their use may entail. Once a pathological label has been applied to an individual, and accepted, his or her expectations and those of significant others change in a way that may make more probable the problematic behaviors or situations under concern (Rosenhan, 1984). Anita, although initially relieved to gain some understanding of her distress, began feeling and acting hopelessly enslaved to an unfulfilling existence. Her husband felt absolved of any responsibility to address the legitimacy of his wife's concerns about their marital relationship. Similarly, the more Lynn monitored her daughter's depression, the more evidence she found to confirm her diagnosis. In both cases, the responses to the labels influenced their continued validity. Anita's husband's efforts to calm her ultimately led to her confirmation of her disorder.

In many ways, this should not be surprising, because it has long been known that elements are given meaning by the context in which they occur. Gestalt psychology has emphasized this point through its elaboration of figure and ground. Asch (1946) has demonstrated that there are central "traits" (such as warm or cold) that are so influential that they significantly color the meaning of other information in forming an impression of another person. Attributions of disorders or dysfunctions are probably among the most powerful of such central traits (Rosenhan, 1984). Once abnormality is ascribed, all other behaviors and characteristics are colored by that label. Nonadherence to the invariant validity of diagnoses and pathological labels challenges the therapist and the client to search for alternative descriptions of the presenting concern that may promote, rather than restrict, change.

Labels of pathology locate the source of the aberration within the individual and only rarely within the complex of interactive sequences and environmental influences that surround the individual's experience of the problem. Anita's diagnosis ignored the complex sequence of events that led to her suicide attempt, and in doing so discounted the validity of her distress. That same process of discounting and invalidation continued when her husband attempted to calm her rather than listen and address her concerns as legitimate.

Diagnoses and labels of pathology assume that there is a *real* problem that exists in some common pattern or redundancy related to some particular kind of real cause (true maintainer). The problem plaguing this assumption is that there is only the vaguest and most general notion of what normal mental health is, while for the diagnosis of pathology, there exists detailed catalogs of deviant behaviors (Watzlawick, 1984).

Other medical specialties that work with catalogs of pathology refer to certain deviations from *well-established* normal functions of the healthy organism. In the mental health field, however, pathology is considered the known factor, and normality is difficult to define. Such a view sets the context for an ongoing therapeutic system of self-fulfilling diagnosis (Watzlawick, 1984).

Self-fulfilling diagnosis results from the selective processing of information that clients present and theoretical expectancies that not only actively influence what information we consider, but also may elicit those very behaviors that confirm our theories. It is our theories or models of human behavior and pathology that interpret client behavior and all the other information we supposedly discover in psychotherapy. The information that the client presents is a result of dynamic social interaction that is influenced by the therapist. Diagnosis, therefore, is not the antiseptically clean and objective endeavor of identifying and cataloguing client concerns, but rather is a therapist-generated meaning that organizes the experience of psychotherapy and confirms the therapist's expectations. Diagnosis and labels of pathology are also responses to the demands of reimbursement/insurance needs and the constraints of the systems in which therapists practice.

Ideally, each client should be accepted as a unique individual with reference to diagnosis as only another way of describing the client's dilemma that may or may not be helpful to consider. We believe that effective psychotherapy *requires* a respect for human complexity that goes well beyond the restricted mentality that accompanies most diagnostic labels.

While it is true that many diagnostic systems and proponents of accurate diagnoses warn against equating the label with the total person, it is difficult, if not impossible, to avoid this extension. Unfortunately, what we often hear are therapists discussing what should be done with "borderlines," "alcoholics," etc., as if those labels *are* the person and actually capture the essence of the diagnosed person's experience of the world. It is unfortunate that useful generalities about specific problem areas are confused with a belief that the generalities themselves represent inherent truths. Viewing and treating an individual as a label disconfirms the complexity and beauty of human variance and discounts the idiosyncratic strengths that so-called abnormal individuals may utilize to live more satisfying lives.

To criticize the notion of pathology and diagnoses in no way is to question the fact that some behaviors are deviant, odd, or self-defeating (Rosenhan, 1984). Sexual abuse of children is deviant; hearing voices is odd. Although we are espousing a health-based view, we are not advocating that a therapist never consider the information that a diagnosis may yield or never use the content of a diagnostic category for discussion in psychotherapy. It is particularly relevant for use if the client holds such a view, and it has proven helpful (e.g., a client who has read a self-help book about co-dependency and has benefited from it).

The information that accompanies diagnostic nomenclature may be attended to by the therapist, but it may never be relevant or utilized as input into the therapeutic conversation or intervention process. For example, a client presenting himself as a messenger from God was arrested for disturbing the peace, because he was awakening strangers in the middle of the night to spread God's word. The therapist considered the diagnostic information from "schizophrenia" as one of many ways to conceptualize the problem that might ultimately be relevant to pursue. However, the client's complaint of being unable to spread God's word was accepted. The therapeutic conversation and intervention were focused on the difficulties inherent in being a messenger from God, rather than on content taken from a psychopathological view of schizophrenia. It is our intent to advocate the pragmatic use of a diagnostic knowledge base without being restricted to sole reliance on it and without such a knowledge base taking any precedence whatsoever over clients' presentations of their concerns.

Summary

The problem attended to by the therapist, then, is not to be found in diagnostic systems. Rather, the problem process, or the *interaction* between the client and others attempting resolution, and the *interaction* between the meaning-constructing client and the social environment is the "problem" attended to by the therapist. The client's content-ordered description of that problem process offers the entry point for intervention. Each problem description, therefore, is unique to the context-based realities of the participants in the problem. The salient features are the idiosyncrasies of the individual involved and the inherent strengths imbedded in those idiosyncrasies, rather than the commonalities that are said to exist in theories of pathology and diagnosis.

Interactional Process:
The Therapist–Client Relationship

To the extent that our emphasis is on the primacy of the client's subjective reality, we are advocating an approach that is phenomenological and client centered in nature. Understanding and respecting the client's meaning system through all phases of treatment is the basis for both the therapeutic relationship and the intervention process. Although considered separately to facilitate discussion, the therapeutic relationship and the intervention process are part and parcel of the same thing. One, the intervention process, is an in-or-out-of-session extension of the other, the therapeutic relationship. Said another way, intervention is an enactment of the interpersonal context set by the therapeutic relationship. We will elaborate on that later, but for now let's look more closely at the relationship separate from intervention processes.

Empathy, Respect, and Genuineness

The common factors (empathy, respect, genuineness) form the core of the therapeutic relationship and are "aspects of psychotherapy and appear to be common elements in a wide variety of approaches to psychotherapy and counseling" (Truax & Carkhuff, 1967, p. 25). All schools of therapy accept the notion that these therapist-provided variables are important for significant progress to occur and are in essence fundamental in the formation of a working alliance (Lambert et al., 1986). Client ratings of therapist understanding, acceptance, and respect have been found to be related positively to outcome across a wide variety of therapies, and such findings are common in the literature. Lambert (1986) suggests that, at least from the client's point of view (which we believe to be the most relevant), effective treatment is due to factors associated with relationship variables and the personal qualities and attitudes of the therapist. Similar findings from the family therapy research literature also emphasize relationship variables. For example, Kuehl, Newfield, and Joanning (1990) found that clients who viewed their therapist as personable, caring, and competent, and as not rigidly adhering to a particular point of view were more likely to be satisfied with their therapeutic experiences.

The notion of the therapeutic relationship, however, is varied and complex. Empathy, respect, and genuineness are themselves a complex set of variables that need more careful definition and analysis so that they may be operationalized more effectively. Patterson (1989) has suggested that more attention should be paid to the client's perceptions—a necessity originally proposed by Rogers—that have not been adequately studied.

The Client's Interpretation

One way of more carefully defining aspects of therapist behavior that empower common factor effects is to extend the definition beyond the therapist's verbal contribution, to include the client's interpretation of the therapist's behavior and the implicit and explicit values and assumptions to which the therapist subscribes. Consider the therapist behavior of empathy. Truax and Carkhuff (1967) define empathy as the therapist's ability to be "accurately empathic, be with the client, be understanding, or grasp the client's meaning," or as the ability to recognize, sense, and understand the feelings that another person has associated with his or her behavior and verbal expressions and to communicate accurately this understanding (Carkhuff, 1971). While the previous definitions describe the therapist's expressed empathy, they do not address the client's idiosyncratic interpretation of the therapist's behavior. Such is the case in much of the research literature addressing outcome and empathy. As Gurman (1977) and Patterson (1984) have argued, the reliance on external ratings of empathy is basically inconsistent with client-centered theory, given the essential importance of the client's perception. We would add that not only are external ratings antithetical to client-centered theory, but also that any rating of empathy other than the client's rating of empathy is virtually irrelevant. After all, therapy is for clients, and their ratings of empathy are powerful indicators of outcome (Gurman, 1977; LaCrosse, 1980; Marziali, 1984). An exception to the client-excluded definition of empathy is provided by

Barrett-Lennard (1981). In his cyclical model of interpersonal empathy, he delineates the phase of the client's experience of the therapist's expressed empathy, which he termed *received empathy*. Preceding received empathy are the two phases of the therapist's resonation of the client's presentation and the communication of empathic understanding.

It is this "received empathy" or the client's perception and experience of the therapist's behavior that is of particular importance. However empathic a therapist may be by the standards of a chosen theoretical orientation, an empathic response may have little or no positive impact on certain clients, or it may be interpreted by some clients as having negative impact (remember Mike and Nancy). The therapist's reliance on standby responses to convey empathy will not be equally productive in terms of the client's perception of being understood. Furthermore, the potential for positive enhancement of common factors will then not occur in those situations in which the therapist's empathic response does not fit the empathic needs of the individual client. Bachelor (1988) provides strong support for this assertion and reached similar conclusions from a research perspective in a recent study examining received empathy. She found that 44% of clients studied perceived their therapist's empathy as cognitive, 30% as affective, 18% as sharing, and 7% as nurturant. Bachelor concluded that empathy has different *meanings* to different clients and should not be viewed or practiced as universal construct.

An Empathic Approach

An approach more consistent with the client's experience would view empathy as a function of the client's unique perception or meaning system and, therefore, would respond flexibly to the client's empathic needs as determined by feedback from the client acquired during the interview process. The interactional effect of the therapist's behavior must be understood in terms of the client's perception or interpretation of that behavior. This interpretation is ultimately determined by the client's unique history and evolving organization of perceptions and experience. The same therapist behavior, be it relationship oriented or intervention oriented, may be interpreted very differently by different clients. When the therapist acts in a way that is consistent with the client's experience of the concern that served as the impetus for therapy, then empathy may be perceived, and common factors beyond the therapist's verbal expression of empathy activated.

Empathy, as perceived by the client, is central to the approach we are espousing: empathy *not* as a specific therapist behavior or attitude (e.g., reflection of feeling is inherently good and empathic); *not* as a means to gain a relationship so that a switch can be made to promote a particular theoretical orientation or therapist personal value; and *not* as a way of teaching clients what a relationship should be. Rather, empathy is therapist attitudes and behaviors that place the client's perceptions and experiences above theoretical content and personal values. Empathy is attempting to understand and *work within* the expressed meaning system of the client.

Respect and Genuineness

Although not as researched and related separately to outcome as empathy, the client's interpretation or perception of therapist respect and genuineness can be similarly viewed as highly idiosyncratic and specific to the unique meaning system of the client. Respect, according to Rogers (1957), means the ability to prize or value the client as a person with worth and dignity. Central to the therapist's behavior of attempting to convey respect is a nonjudgmental attitude that allows for the avoidance of condemnation of the client's actions or motives and acceptance of the client's expressions and experiences (Rogers, 1957).

Operationalizing respect entails embracing a nonpathological and nonpejorative perspective of people that necessarily assumes that *all* clients can make more satisfying lives for themselves and have the inherent capacity to do so. We believe that the antithesis of respect may be the attribution of pathology that suggests a negative outcome. Respect may also be operationalized by having no particular theoretical ax to grind with clients. Interpretations made to clients or meanings imposed by therapists despite the clients' lack of acceptance or acknowledgment are disrespectful. Respect for the client is assured, and the dignity of the client is promoted when a therapist discards a particular interpretation or meaning if the client deems it unacceptable or unhelpful. Again, it is the client's perception and the therapist's ability to be sensitive to the client's input regarding the acceptability of any therapist behavior that constitutes respect. The Kuehl et al. (1990) study supports a respectful stance by their finding that clients prefer therapists who do not rigidly adhere to a particular point of view. The authors suggest that therapists should proceed cautiously when trying to convince a client of the utility or rightness of an approach the client does not readily accept.

Genuineness means being oneself without being "phony." Therapists who do not overemphasize their role, authority, or status are more likely to be perceived as more genuine by clients (Cormier & Cormier, 1991). From our perspective, genuineness is embodied in the therapist's adoption of an honest cautiousness and tentativeness about approaching the client, conceptualizing his or her concerns, and intervening to address those concerns. A genuine tentativeness in the therapist's presentation when the therapist provides input into the problem process conveys to the client

TABLE 3.1. Therapist-Provided Variables

Therapist behavior	Definition
Empathy	Attitudes and behaviors that place the client's perception and experience above the theoretical content and personal values; empathy is manifested by the therapist's attempts to not only accept and assume the internal frame of reference of the client, but more important, to work within the expressed meaning system of the client.
Respect	Attitudes and behaviors that place the value of the client as a person with worth and dignity above pejorative, pathological, or theoretical perspectives; respect is manifested by therapist sensitivity to the acceptability of any therapist behavior to the client's meaning system.
Genuineness	Attitudes and behaviors that avoid phoniness and an overemphasis on authority, and embody an honest cautiousness regarding approaching the client, conceptualizing the client's concerns, and intervening to address those concerns; genuineness is manifested by an acceptance of the lack of definitive understanding provided by psychotherapy theory.
Validation	An individualized combination of the therapist-provided variables; the therapist genuinely accepts the client's presentation at face value, the therapist respects the client's experience of the problem by highlighting its importance, and the therapist empathically offers total justification of the client's experience.
Operationalizing common factors	Accomplished by the therapist's adoption of the client's meaning system as his or her theoretical orientation, thereby allowing the client's idiosyncratic experience of the world to become the guiding theory that dictates therapist behavior.

that the therapist claims no corner on reality and is not the deliverer of truth, but rather is a collaborator who, because of training and experience, can offer hopefully productive input. The therapist genuinely holds that the client is indeed the expert regarding the concern that served as the impetus for therapy and acts accordingly. We believe that phoniness is exemplified by the position that holds theories of psychotherapy and their application to client concerns as being the way things really are, rather than one of many best guesses or approximations. Being authentic may require a humbling acceptance of the nondefinitive nature of the profession of psychotherapy and the inherent complexity of human beings.

Table 3.1 defines the therapist-provided variables and summarizes the bottom-line point that organizes our perceptions and experience regarding operationalizing common factors: The client's meaning system

is the theoretical orientation adopted by the therapist. From that acceptance, the client's frame of reference becomes the guiding theory that
dictates therapist actions/interventions.

Validation

Operationalizing common factors is also accomplished by a therapist's
verbal behavior called *validation*. Validation is a therapist-initiated process
in which the client's thoughts, feelings, and behaviors are accepted,
believed, and considered completely understandable, given the client's
subjective experience of the world. Validation represents a combined
expression of empathy, respect, and genuineness that is individually
tailored to the idiosyncracies of the client's experience. The therapist
genuinely accepts the client's presentation at face value and holds the
belief that the client is doing the best that he or she can, the therapist
respects the client's experience of the problem by emphasizing its importance, and the therapist empathically offers total justification of the
client's experience. The therapist, therefore legitimizes the client's meaning system, and in the process may replace the invalidation that may be a
part of it.

The therapist accepted Lynn's view of her daughter's genetic depression at face value and legitimized that view in the presentation of the
diathesis-stress model. Lynn's attempts at helping her daughter were
justified as understandable and appropriate, and as reflective of Lynn's
obvious love and concern for her daughter. Anita's perspective of BPD was
similarly accepted and legitimized in the therapist's pursuit of Anita's
childhood experiences. As therapy unfolded, many opportunities arose to
justify Anita's feelings regarding her husband's tightfisted control over
finances and his habitual yielding to his parents' desires. Validating
Anita's concerns seemed to replace the invalidation present in her
husband's behavior, as well as the diagnosis of BPD. Validation seemed to
allow both Lynn and Anita to risk a revision of meaning about their
concerns.

Common factors, therefore, are expressed through the acceptance of
the client's meaning system as the guiding theory and by the validation of
that meaning system. Common factors are further manifested by specific
interventions that convey or implement therapist validation.

Relationship and Technique

The growing evidence of the importance of the relationship may lead
some to conclude that intervention or technique is less important than
the relationship aspects of therapy. However, as alluded to earlier,
relationship and intervention factors are interdependent aspects of the

same process. The actions or techniques that the therapist may use to intervene are intrinsically linked to the interpersonal context in which they occur. Butler and Strupp (1986) argue:

> The complexity and subtlety of psychotherapeutic process cannot be reduced to a set of disembodied techniques, because the techniques gain their meaning, and in turn, their effectiveness, from the particular interaction of the individuals involved. (p. 33)

The interactional context that creates meaning for intervention are the characteristics, attitudes, and behaviors of the therapist that provide the core conditions as perceived by the client. Common factors are manifested by specific interventions that *convey* or *implement* the therapist's understanding and acceptance of the client's meaning system.

For example, consider the technique of symptom prescription. Asking a client to engage in the problem that brought him or her to therapy must emerge from meanings generated in the therapeutic interaction. The prescription may gain meaning for the client following a mutual exploration of the complexities involved in the problem and an authentic desire by the therapist to learn more about the problem. Furthermore, the so-called prescription must also represent an extension of the core conditions or be perceived by the client as somehow conveying the therapist's understanding and respect for his or her experience of the world. The prescription may validate the experience of the client who thinks that the problem has been trivialized by others and feels ashamed and incompetent because of the inability to control or handle the problem. If the technique is offered without a contextual meaning or does not demonstrate the therapist's understanding, it is unlikely to be effective and may even be harmful.

This brief example illustrates that the variety of outcomes that may result from a given technique or intervention are primarily a function of the interpersonal and meaning context surrounding the intervention. The effectiveness of the intervention depends on the meaning the client ascribes to it, and that meaning is acquired in the interactional context of the therapist and client. Technique and relationship are completely interdependent and cannot be separated. *Intervention, then, becomes the behavioral manifestation of the relationship.* Intervention in the form of tasks or assignments extends the interpersonal context defined in session to the client's social environment.

Successful psychotherapy emerges from neither relationship nor technique factors. Proponents of "relationship only" perspectives rarely discuss clients that do not respond to the model's perspective of the core conditions. Proponents of specific techniques aimed at particular disorders always presuppose an acceptable level of client cooperation

(Butler & Strupp, 1986). What appears to matter the most from our point of view is the therapist's ability to flexibly accommodate a wide variety of client interpersonal styles and meaning systems. This is achieved through sensitivity to the client's perception of the core conditions, a genuine acceptance and validation of the client's meaning system, and an extension of that common factors context to the client's social environment through the intervention process. The thought of skillfully managing such a complex and difficult task has been a very humbling experience.

Discussion of the relative importance of relationship and technique will likely continue. Another way to understand their interaction in therapy is provided by the concept of the working alliance, which we will discuss here.

2. THE CLIENT'S PRESENTATION, RATHER THAN THE THERAPIST'S ORIENTATION, DETERMINES THERAPY GOALS, THE CONTENT OF THE THERAPEUTIC CONVERSATION, AND INTERVENTION STRATEGIES

It is the client's construction of meaning around the problem that is of importance to the problem process, as well as to the intervention selected. Assessment focuses on establishing a consensual understanding of the complaint from the client's perspective. It is the client's presentation of the problem that establishes the entry point for change. "Presentation" involves the client's verbal and nonverbal description of and beliefs regarding the nature and meaning of the complaint as well as the affective experience that attends the problem. Therapeutic interaction involves a systematic mutual exploration and definition of the meanings and experiences associated with the client's presenting concern. Exploration of the concern and its meaning requires a candid exchange between the therapist and client, as well as a collaborative formulation of outcome criteria that are specified by the client. The therapist may offer ideas for discussion that grow into relevant dialogue or fade away as it becomes apparent that they are not meaningful for the client to pursue. Collaboration is dependent upon the client's agreement with what problems will be worked on, criteria for successful improvement or resolution of the problem, and methods used to address the problems.

Therapy then, seeks to create a conversational context that allows for mutual collaboration in the problem-defining and problem-revising processes. The client's judgment regarding experiences that are relevant for discussion and intervention is respected. Clients are, in essence, in "charge" of the content, while therapists are in "charge" of the process of unfolding that content.

The Therapeutic Alliance

Let us emphasize the importance of mutual goal definition and collaborative formulation of treatment methods through a discussion of the concept of therapeutic alliance. The therapeutic alliance (hereafter referred to just as "alliance") has been viewed by many as the quintessential integrative variable because its importance does not lie within the specifications or content of any one school of thought. The alliance speaks to a *process* of psychotherapy or a method of securing a client's cooperation and commitment to therapy. Although the primary theoretical and empirical work on the alliance has come from psychodynamic and Rogerian perspectives, there has recently been a growing recognition of the role of the alliance in other psychotherapy approaches. These developments have contributed to a view of the centrality of the alliance in the change process of a variety of approaches, even if the latter are heterogeneous with respect to the proposed mechanism of change.

Bordin (1979) formulated three interacting components of the alliance: (1) agreement on the goals of psychotherapy; (2) agreement on the tasks of psychotherapy (specific techniques, topics of conversation, interview procedures, frequency of meeting); and (3) the development of a relationship bond between the therapist and client. The therapeutic alliance, then, is comprised of the common-factor effects discussed previously and is a function of the degree of agreement between the therapist and client about the goals and tasks of psychotherapy. While the bonding dimension reiterates the importance of the relationship and its affective qualities, the agreement on goals and tasks refers to the more cognitive aspects by focusing on the congruence between the client's and the therapist's beliefs about how people change in therapy. Supporting our earlier assertion that technique must flow from the meaning system of the client, Bordin (1979) suggests that the effectiveness of any therapeutic technique depends on the vividness with which the therapist links the intervention strategy to the client's difficulty and ideas of how he or she wants to or can change.

Empirical evidence supports the direct association between the alliance and outcome, especially the alliance as rated in the early phase of therapy (Bachelor, 1991; Hartley & Strupp, 1983; Horvath & Greenberg, 1986; Luborsky, Crits-Christoph, Alexander, Margolis, & Cohen, 1983). In the family therapy literature, similar findings have emerged. Pinsof and Catherall (1986) developed alliance scales for use in family therapy research and have demonstrated that higher scores on the scales correlate significantly with therapist ratings of improvement in couple and family therapy.

Suffice it to say that therapist imposition of goals or tasks may not be conducive to successful outcome. It may also be interpreted as disrespectful and, therefore, may not enhance common factors. Lynn's goal for therapy was to help Amy with her depression via the therapist's active suggestions regarding how she might help. Anita's goal was to understand her BPD through pursuit of her childhood experiences. The therapist accepted the client's goals and respected the client's view about how therapy should pursue those goals.

Selection of Content

In addition to the agreement of goals and tasks (i.e., respecting the client's meaning system about the desired change and the means to such change), the actual *content* of the therapeutic conversation should similarly be agreed upon and fit the client's experience of the problem. This process also requires a mutual exchange of ideas in which the therapist receives feedback from the client regarding any content formulation that the therapist may offer.

Therapist allegiance to any particular theoretical content involves a trade-off that simultaneously enables and restricts intervention options. Process-oriented therapists walk a tightrope, balancing themselves between the flexibility and uncertainty of process and the directionality and limitations of content (Held, 1986). Because a process-oriented approach focuses on changing the interaction that maintains the complaint or concern, establishing "The One True Reality" is neither a function nor a goal.

A purpose of the therapeutic conversation is to make explicit the client's reality related to the problem process. The content of the therapeutic conversation provides a meaningful framework that may allow the client to reorganize perception and experience, thus shifting the problem-enabling meaning system. The therapist may respond to the client's complaint with content selected from a number of sources: (1) generic response patterns; (2) specific clinical content areas and techniques; and (3) specific theoretical or philosophical orientations. The therapist may also respond with content arising *solely* from the client's description and not introduce any other content.

Sources of Content

Generic response patterns (e.g., the grief process, Kubler-Ross, 1969; rape trauma syndrome, Burgess & Holmstrom, 1979, etc.) describe culturally typical patterns or phases of response to developmental transitions or incidental crises, and may provide the basis for an intervention strategy that shifts the meaning system surrounding the problematic response. Likewise, content derived from a specific clinical area (e.g., anxiety, AIDS, etc.) may provide an organizing framework for the therapeutic conversation and intervention. This new information may provide a reorganization of the solution patterns or a rationale for intervention.

Sometimes clients present with discrete, clearly delineated concerns. With some complaints, the literature strongly indicates the efficacy of a *particular approach, specific conceptualization, or technique* (e.g., perform-ance anxiety, relaxation training, symptom prescription). Attending to the literature and selecting interventions associated with documented, successful outcomes serves the client by extending the options for intervention and enhancing therapeutic flexibility. Content drawn from this source may be utilized as a primary framework for intervention or as an adjunct to other interventions (Duncan & Parks, 1988).

Regardless of how well the selected content (technique) is supported by research, tradition, and/or clinical literature, client acceptance of this therapist-introduced content is the critical variable. Selected content is virtually useless if clients do not view it as applicable or helpful to their particular circumstances.

Consider a client presenting with a simple phobia. Consulting the literature suggests that the treatment of choice is behavioral and requires structured, consistent, exposure-based exercises (Barlow, 1988). Such techniques are successful with 75% of clients with phobias (Barlow & Wolfe, 1981). However, an examination of the results of this and other studies reveals that an average of 25% of clients dropped out and were not included in the outcome data. If dropouts are included, success rates drop to 50% (Prochaska, 1991).

This may indicate that while behavioral techniques for phobias are worthwhile, such techniques must also be congruent with, and demonstrate acceptance of, the client's meaning system. In other words, such techniques must also flow from the common factors context of the therapeutic relationship. The selection of technique or content, therefore, must go beyond the mere prescriptive matching of client problems with research-demonstrated techniques.

Should the client's presentation appear congruent with a *particular theoretical orientation*, the therapist may utilize that content to introduce different meanings to the conversation and construct interventions. Presenting the concern in the language of a particular approach (e.g., discussing client complaints of depression, malaise, and meaninglessness from an existential perspective) may enable a reorganization of the meaning system that supports the problem process.

The selection of content is not data based or empirically driven and is not directed by a concrete prescriptive specificity because the matching decision operates at a level of abstraction that views content as analogical. Content is selected for its congruence or complementarity to the client's world view and circumstances, rather than the theoretical predilection of the therapist. Content is only the vehicle through which the problem process is influenced. While the content matching decision is not determined by diagnosis, symptom complexity, client coping style (Beutler, 1986), or any other *content-based decision trees*, intervention may incorporate any of these factors. The matching decision is based entirely in the content-laden description of the presenting concern offered by the client and the emergent process of the therapist–client conversation. Therefore, any client or problem quality could be relevant if directed by the idiosyncratic content focus of the client.

Lynn's perception of "genetic depression" served as the impetus for the selection of the diathesis-stress formulation (a specific clinical content area). The content, therefore, was client directed. Anita's content presentation regarding BPD focused the therapeutic conversation such that no other formal content area was introduced by the therapist. In both cases, the content of the conversation was directed by the idiosyncratic content description provided by the client and emerged from the interview process.

3. INTERVENTION INTERRUPTS THE PROBLEM CYCLE, PROVIDES MEANING REVISION OPPORTUNITIES, AND VALIDATES THE CLIENT'S EXPERIENCE

This assumption addresses how intervention provides a context for clients to change the problem or circumstance that served as the impetus for therapy. Intervention promotes change at three, hierarchically nested, descriptive levels.

The first level of change describes intervention as enabling an interruption of the behavioral interaction that constitutes the problem cycle. In MRI terms, this is the interdiction of repetitively misapplied solution attempts of the client and others with whom he or she interacts. This description of change views strategy or technique as deliberate therapeutic attempts to influence the client to simply "do something different" (de Shazer, 1985) regarding the presenting problem. Intervention is said to jam the problem cycle so that a new cycle of behavioral interaction can ensue. Interruption of the problem cycle also creates an opportunity for meaning revision and is, therefore, subsumed under the second level of change.

From the second level of description of the change process, intervention provides meaning revision opportunities, either in the client's interactive experience of the problem, or in the interview process itself. Meaning revision in the client's interactive experience of the problem is promoted by suggestions by the therapist that enable a behavioral, cognitive, or affective competition with the client's current experience of the problem. Meaning revision in the interview process involves the conversational recreation of the client's experience and the collaborative generation of new or altered meanings.

Altering Interactional Experience

Individuals continually generate, confirm, challenge, and revise meaning as they interact in the social environment. Intervention entails suggesting changes in the interactional context or what the client and others are *doing*, *thinking*, and/or *feeling* regarding the situation or experiences the client defined as problematic, thereby promoting the possibility for the client to challenge the limits of their constructed meanings. Placing clients and the problem process in a different context creates a situation through which new meaning may be ascribed (Erickson, 1980), as well as interrupts the current problem-maintaining solution attempts.

Interventions directed toward altering the interactional experience involve the therapist's suggestion of *competing experiences*. This class of interventions includes tasks, prescriptions, direct suggestions, and homework assignments; each strategy attempts to set up the interactional process surrounding the problem so that the problem cycle is interrupted, and clients may independently resolve the dilemma that brought them to therapy.

The new context enabled by competing experiences competes in a behavioral, cognitive, or affective way with the client's current experience of the problem. Competition with the different components of the client's meaning system permits a revision of the client's experience of the problem and, therefore, perhaps an emergent meaning system that is less distressing. Such a competition enables clients to challenge the limitations of their operative meaning systems and permits a revision of the meaning system in vivo, thereby perhaps empowering spontaneous remission effects.

Spontaneous remission may be viewed not as truly spontaneous, but rather as one possible result of a competing meaning experience. The revised meaning allows for alternative solutions to the problem, thereby resulting in new meanings, etc. The therapist only suggests a change in the context or interactional process; change in the meaning system occurs in the course of the actual interaction.

Lynn

The intervention with Lynn is an example of a competing experience. It was specifically designed to promote a revision opportunity in the client's interactive experience of the problem. The therapist directly suggested that Lynn back off, lessen her involvement in her daughter's everyday activities, and allow her daughter to work through and learn to cope with her depression. The therapist suggested that Lynn could facilitate the process of working through by encouraging expression of Amy's concerns, validating them, and even exaggerating them, rather than acting upon them.

Such a competing *behavioral* experience may result in a change of contingencies surrounding the problem, enabling new or different behaviors to occur in place of the old problematic ones. The competing behaviors may generate the construction of a new meaning system that does not include the presenting complaint; the particular change in meaning is constructed by the client's behaviorally altered interaction with the environment. Lynn accepted the therapist's suggestions and returned for two more sessions. She reported that her daughter seemed happier and was complaining less. Lynn also said that although it was difficult for her, she was not attempting to rescue Amy from her depression any more and that perhaps her daughter was only mildly predisposed to depression. Lynn's solution attempts were interrupted and she revised her meaning of Amy's genetic depression such that Lynn no longer believed antidepressant medication was needed.

Revising Meaning in Session

While competing experiences are indirectly related to meaning in that the attempt is to change the context, meaning revision interventions seek direct alteration, replacement, or empowerment of a particular meaning system. Because individuals can recall and review an interaction following its termination and continue to organize their perceptions and experience, acquired meaning systems can be influenced apart from the actual transaction. Meaning can be influenced via the ongoing dialogue that occurs in psychotherapy.

Direct exploration of the client's perceptions and experiences associated with the complaint may promote the construction of alternate ascriptions by the client or the therapist. These emergent meanings are cogenerated and mutually formulated in that they arise from the therapeutic conversation and include input from both the client and the therapist. Meaning revision strategies, although differentiated into client and therapist ascribed for descriptive purposes, represent the culmination of a meaningful exchange between the therapist and client. This class of interventions includes *empowering client ascribed meaning* and *ascribing different meanings to problem situations*.

Because of the ongoing nature of meaning generation, meaning formation and the understanding of any phenomenon are always interpretive processes and are open for input and revision. There are no fixed and uniquely correct meanings or interpretations that run across situations or problems that clients bring to therapy, nor are there any inherently right ways to describe or direct the therapeutic conversation. As mind-boggling as it sounds and perhaps as frightening as it feels, such a view opens unlimited possibilities for change and growth. One way of enacting this view is to follow the client's lead regarding the content of the conversation and to allow therapy to be a process of expanding and unfolding the client's meaning and experience, thereby actually creating new meanings for those experiences (Anderson & Goolishian, 1988). From this perspective, therapy is a process that seeks to create a context for new meanings to develop and to be ascribed by the client and therapist.

Reexperiencing and Reconstructing Memories

A major support of the significance of the interview process itself to meaning revision comes from the experimental literature regarding memory. Memory can no longer be thought of as an archival system of specific memories or complete records of discrete episodes, but rather as a process involving bits and pieces of information that are continually interpreted and reconstructed during the course of remembering. Memories, and the meanings attached to them, are not static, but are constantly evolving recreations; they are not discrete units linked up over time, but instead are a dynamically changing system (Rosenfield, 1988). Clients relating their experiences to the therapist, therefore, are reconstructing those experiences each time, such that the possibility for the generation of a different, more helpful meaning is always present.

Spence (1984) suggests that the process of the client providing information to the therapist during the course of therapy results, not in the uncovering of objective facts or historical truth, but rather in the generation of an articulated narrative understanding or narrative truth. This perspective, which is very consistent with the Goolishian and Anderson (1987) perspective of language-based systems, posits the therapist role as assisting the client in an articulation of narrative truth by gradually organizing the information into a consistent portrait. A continuous process of revision takes place in which a "new" articulation of the narrative truth emerges as a product of the communication between the therapist and the client (Shafer, 1983).

The therapeutic conversation promotes the emergence of new or

revised meaning through the exploration of the experiences and perceptions that the client chooses to articulate. Therapy, then, is a meaning
revision process in which each articulation of the client's concerns
presents an opportunity for a different experience of those concerns.

Anita

Continual exploration of Anita's narrative regarding the sequence of
events that led to her suicide attempt permitted an ongoing possibility for
meaning revision. Each time Anita articulated her experiences, the
diagnosis of BPD seemed to lose credibility, and other explanations
seemed to become more plausible. For example, as she remembered the
precipitating fight with her husband regarding their holiday schedule
with his parents, Anita expressed her feelings and perceptions about her
husband's propensity for acquiescing to his parent's wishes.

Following several discussions in which Anita expressed misgivings
about her diagnosis, as well as articulated other experiences related to the
suicide attempt, the therapist "intervened" with the question regarding
the accuracy of the diagnosis. After exploring what that meant, Anita
asked what the therapist thought her diagnosis really should be. The
therapist responded to the client's question and her desire for a diagnosis
with "some therapists may say that perhaps a diagnosis of dysthymic
disorder would be more accurate." The therapist's ascription of a different
meaning arose from the ongoing process of meaning revision that was
enabled by the client's articulation of her experiences. The revised
meaning for the client's experience continued to unfold and expand; the
client's emphasis on her diagnosis ultimately led her to question its
validity and empowered her to address the unsatisfying aspects of her life.
Anita secured a part-time job, took an interior design class, and
convinced her husband to enter marital therapy. The client experienced
a meaning revision from something outside of her control to something
she could proactively address.

The distinction between competing experiences and meaning
revision interventions is somewhat arbitrary, given the inherent
reciprocity of meaning and behavior and the necessary connection
between in-session and out-of-session intervention. The distinction
represents an attempt to delineate avenues by which the client's
experience of the concerns that served as the impetus for therapy may be
influenced and illustrates the salient features of the different strategies.

Intervention and Validation

Intervention has been discussed as providing interruptions of the problem
cycle and as promoting revision opportunities. The third level of change

describes intervention as also providing a way to extend the common factors context of the relationship to the client's social environment. Intervention can enable an in vivo validation of the client's meaning system, thereby supporting the client in revising the problem experience. Intervention, then, is an explicit therapist behavior that demonstrates empathy, respect, and genuineness, and directly validates the client's experience of the world.

Accepting Lynn's meaning system regarding her daughter's genetic depression, rather than confronting it or attempting to persuade Lynn to change her view, enabled the therapist to make a suggestion based upon the genetic depression meaning. The intervention itself demonstrated therapist empathy and respect for Lynn's perspective of Amy's depression, and promoted the alliance because the client's goals were accepted, and the suggestion directly addressed those goals.

Said another way, the intervention was congruent with Lynn's meaning system in that the suggestion was made *because* Lynn's daughter had a genetic depression. Interventions that are designed as suggestions based in the client's meaning system are inherently validating because the intervention demonstrates the therapist's acceptance of the client's meaning each time the client enacts the suggestion. Each time a suggestion is attempted, the alliance is extended to the client's natural world. Each time Lynn encouraged, validated, and exaggerated her daughter's negative expressions, she did so in service of helping Amy with her genetic depression. The competing experience interrupted Lynn's solutions of cheering and reassurance, it created an opportunity for meaning revision through Lynn's behaviorally altered interaction, and it validated Lynn's meaning of genetic depression. Validation, once experienced, may allow clients the support and freedom to risk a revision of meaning about their concerns. Out-of-session validation is very powerful and perhaps may be the most important aspect of encouraging clients to utilize their own strengths to resolve problems.

SUMMARY AND CONCLUSIONS

To summarize this chapter and highlight our major points, consider the following case example introduced earlier in this chapter:

Joe, a 19-year-old college student, became increasingly preoccupied with religion, the preoccupation culminating in an announcement to his family that he was a messenger from God. Parental attempts to reason calmly with Joe evoked accusations that his parents were "disciples of the devil." When Joe began pounding on doors at all hours, attempting to spread the Word, he was taken into custody. The parents were very invested in avoiding a hospitalization because of the father's very negative experience with a psychiatric hospital many years before.

Assumption #1: The Problem, and Its Solution, Is Embedded in the Interactive Process

Joe's desire to spread God's Word was neither discounted nor pathologized. The problem was viewed as part of the interaction between Joe and others attempting to help him and between Joe's constructed meanings and the social environment. Joe's parents had met Joe's pronouncement with efforts to reason with him and essentially make him see that he wasn't a messenger and that he needed help. Their solution attempts, which were characterized by honest efforts to help Joe, were perceived as discounting his status and subverting his mission. Joe's constructed meaning of his messenger status was viewed as continually evolving and, therefore, open for cogeneration of a revised meaning.

Regardless of possible brain dysfunction/biochemical imbalance, the therapist assumed that an interactional process surrounding the problem would enable therapeutic participation in problem definition and problem solution. Again, we are not suggesting that biochemical imbalances do not exist or do not merit consideration, but rather that sole reliance on such a view restricts options and may preclude therapist collaboration in the construction of a more helpful, problem-improving meaning.

Joe's meaning system was not rejected or discounted; rather, the difficulty he was encountering spreading the Word was explicitly and empathically accepted and validated by the therapist. Joe was accepted as a human being deserving acceptance and validation like any other client. Joe was respected by the therapist and, therefore, was neither confronted nor patronized. The therapist considered Joe's meaning system the theory from which he worked and, therefore, concerned himself with understanding and working within that meaning system.

Assumption #2: The Client's Presentation, Rather Than the Therapist's Orientation, Determines Therapy Goals, the Content of the Therapeutic Conversation, and Intervention Strategies

It was Joe's construction of meaning related to the presenting concern that was viewed as primary to goal formulation, the content of the conversation, and the interventions selected. An exploration of Joe's dilemma resulted in a mutual formulation of a goal for Joe to spread God's word without interference from those who did not understand his mission. The therapist acknowledged Joe's belief that he was called by God, and the problems related to such a calling were discussed. An ongoing dialogue ensued, and the therapist suggested that the power of God's message might appear frightening, confusing, and overwhelming to the unenlightened, thus leading many to discount and retreat from Joe's intended efforts to share God's message of love. The content of Joe's meaning system provided the vehicle through which new meaning emerged in the session as well as formed the basis for the therapist to suggest a competing experience. Consider the following abbreviated dialogue and ensuing therapist suggestion of a competing experience.

C: I know you won't believe this, but I'm a messenger from God and I have a mission to spread His word to everyone on earth. Do you believe me—that I'm a messenger from God?

T: I believe you and I feel honored to be talking with you, but I'm concerned that no one will hear your very important message.

C: I think I see what you're getting at. You mean that they won't believe me.

T: Yes, and also, that this kind of message is so powerful and divine that it is probably just plain overwhelming to most people who are unenlightened and have not received divine inspiration as you have. I'm afraid that given this, they can't possibly understand the beauty and glory of your message from Him. What scares me is that they will become frightened and confused and will discount the message of love that you're trying to deliver. What do you think?

C: Well, I think you're right.

T: I wonder how else you can spread God's word in more subtle, yet powerful, ways that mere mortals can understand and accept. One thing that occurs to me is that you could possibly share the Word and accomplish your mission on earth by giving God's love to people a little at a time. You could smile His holy smile and greet people with His love and demonstrate His word by your deeds, rather than your words.

Assumption #3 : Intervention Interrupts the Problem Cycle, Provides Meaning Revision Opportunities, and Validates the Client's Experience

After the acceptance of the client's meaning system and an agreement on the goals, a cogenerated meaning emerged regarding the frightening and overwhelming aspects of Joe's attempts to spread the Word. Utilizing Joe's meaning system as the theory from which he operated, as well as the revised meaning regarding the power of the message, the therapist suggested a competing behavioral experience. The different behaviors (e.g., greeting, smiling) thereby changed how Joe interacted with the social environment and vice versa. Joe's parents were encouraged to validate Joe's mission and support his desire to spread the Word. A change in the actual interaction resulted in a change in the contingencies surrounding Joe's mission, thereby allowing for new meaning to be constructed. Over time, Joe constructed a revised meaning concerning his religious beliefs that did not include his special messenger status. Instead, he returned to college two quarters later and pursued a major in religion.

The intervention can be described as interrupting Joe's solution attempts to spread God's word, as well as his parent's solution attempts to help him back to reality (Level One). This interdiction of the problem cycle enabled the start of a different pattern of interaction that did not include the problem. Another way of describing the intervention is that the suggested behavior change competed with Joe's current experience of spreading God's word, thereby enabling Joe to revise his meaning system regarding his messenger status. His behaviorally altered interaction created a context for alternative meanings to be ascribed (Level Two).

Finally, the intervention extended the in-session validation of Joe's meaning system to the outside social environment, therefore continuing to validate Joe's perceptions and experience (Level Three). Each time Joe smiled His holy smile, his experience was validated. The therapist's empathy with Joe's experience created the context for Joe to arrive at a revised meaning independent of the therapist. Common factors effects were highlighted through the therapist's explicit recognition of Joe's meaning system as hierarchically superior to any content-based theoretical frame of reference. Working within that context fostered Joe's identification with the therapist and the development of the alliance, which encouraged Joe to continue in therapy and risk a revision of meaning. At this level of description, intervention based in the client's meaning system implicitly enhanced the effect of common factor variables and directly validated his experience of the world. Accepting Joe allowed him to expect that his new ways of conveying the Word would be heard by others. Joe's changes in conveyance of the Word led to an ultimate return to college.

4 ▨ Initial Interviewing: Describing the Problem, Revising Its Meaning, and Validating the Client's Experience

I NTERVIEWING is not distinct from intervention, just as it is not separate from the therapeutic relationship. Interviewing is not directed toward describing an unchanging entity or assessing a situation that exists in total objective reality. Rather, interviewing is the therapist's participation in a constantly changing process of describing the problem, revising its meaning, and validating the client's experience. Interviewing is also the therapeutic construction of change opportunities through conversation. Therapist sensitivity to these emerging opportunities provides an ongoing possibility for problem resolution.

This chapter presents a practical interview format designed to construct opportunities for client change at three levels. From the description that views strategy as interrupting the behavioral interaction that constitutes the problem cycle, the interview format is designed to elicit information regarding the vicious cycle of unsuccessful solution attempts surrounding the presenting problem. This interactive description of the problem process allows for the design of an intervention to interdict that problem process and permit an alternative solution.

The information-eliciting aspect is couched within the second level (description) of change, which views strategy as promoting meaning revision in the therapy session through the conversational recreation of the client's experience, or out of session in the client's interactive experience of the problem. The information-eliciting format is a vehicle through which meaning unfolds, and opportunities arise for the collaborative generation of new or altered meanings. Seeking information is therefore inherently interventive; questions are not only after answers, but also meaning revision.

This meaning unfolding, exploring, and revision process is itself embedded within a larger context, the third level of change, which views strategy as an extension of the therapist–client relationship. From this overarching context, interviewing seeks to construct opportunities for change through explicit therapist behaviors that demonstrate empathy, respect, and genuineness. This larger relationship frame of reference suggests that eliciting information is not only inherently interventive, but more important, is itself a way of conveying specific common factors by validating the client's experience of the world.

This chapter examines these hierarchically nested, but distinct, descriptive levels of change and suggests that simultaneous consideration of them results in multiple avenues of promoting change. It is the quest for opportunities that arise from the three levels that defines the nature of the initial interview. Because of these ever-present opportunities, every session, including the first interview, presents the possibility that the presenting complaint will be resolved within the session.

DESCRIBING THE PROBLEM

What is first sought is a concrete, action-oriented description, specifically addressing the MRI question, "*Who* is doing *what* that presents a problem, to *whom*, and *how* does such behavior constitute a problem?" (Fisch et al., 1982, p. 70). Additionally, a workable goal is needed, as well as an explanation of why the individual, couple, or family has sought treatment now rather than previously.

It is best for the therapist to adopt a "help me to understand" attitude to a radical degree. Perhaps thinking of oneself as an alien from another planet who will never completely understand is a good way to characterize the attitude we believe to be the most helpful. In essence, the therapist *is* an alien trying to make sense of the client's world of idiosyncratically formed meaning and unique style of communication. It is a complex and ever-changing world that is beyond a definitive understanding. In service of pursuing an interactional description of the problem, the MRI's basic elements of a first interview are well suited: the nature of the complaint, how the problem is being handled, and the client's minimal goals.

Nature of the Complaint

The key words in this phase of the interview are understanding and describing. Generally, the process can begin with, "What brings you here to see me today?" This is preferred over asking what problem brings the client, because the word *problem* can connote something quite different to the client and may impose a "problem" on a situation in which the client may not have previously perceived it as a problem. For example, the client's view may be that it is a dilemma, complaint, or even an idea or decision to discuss and not a problem at all. While such attention to words may seem like overkill, and it may be in many instances, the language that the therapist imposes on the process warrants consideration and should be subject to scrutiny. The point being that the therapist wants to allow for as much space as possible for the client's words and interpretations to emerge, instead of the therapist's. We will return to this aspect of the first interview in the next section, but bear this notion in mind as you continue.

Obtaining the client's description of the nature of the complaint requires a dogged pursuit of the details of the problematic situation. The therapist attempts to elicit information that is clear, explicit, and in behavioral terms; that is, what each individual involved in the problem process is specifically saying and doing in *performing* the problem, rather than general statements or abstract explanations. Requesting examples is often the best way to get specific behavioral descriptions of the client's complaint (Fisch et al., 1982).

Unless the therapist can make a clear statement conveying all the elements of the presenting problem (who, what, to whom, and how), there is not adequate information to design an intervention. Recall that from the level of change that views strategy as interrupting the problem cycle, it follows that a clear description of the problem itself is critical to intervention design. The therapist may consider that an adequate account of the problem has been obtained when he or she can visualize the interactional sequences in which the problem is embedded (Coyne, 1986).

Some clients may give clear and direct answers readily without much prompting, while others will respond in more vague, general, or tangential ways. It is necessary for the therapist to be persistent at times, but always from the genuine attitude that it's the therapist's first experience in the client's world, rather than the client's problem of inarticulation. The therapist accepts that a complete understanding of the client's experience is never possible, but rather attempts to gain closer approximations of it. Table 4.1 presents questions that help to obtain information about the nature of the complaint.

Although what specifically the problem is, of course, is important, how the problem constitutes a problem is more so. How a situation is a problem may often be plain—but is it really? Consider depression. What does it mean to the client? What is the client depressed about? How is the depression a problem? Is it a sleep problem, a performance problem, a

TABLE 4.1. Questions Regarding the Nature of the Complaint and Exceptions to the Problem

---

What brings you here today?
How or in what ways is it a problem?
Can you give me a recent example?
If I were a fly on the wall, what would I see?
If I were doing a documentary about this problem and followed you around with a video camera, what would it look like?
What happens? Then what happens? Then what?
What concerns you most about it?
When does it occur? Where does it occur?
How often does it occur?
How long does it last?
What stops it?
Who is present when the problem happens?
What are they doing or saying?
When doesn't the problem occur?
When is it just a little better?
What are the things occurring in your life right now that you would like to see continue?
Has anything changed for the better since you called for the appointment?
How is it different from when the problem is occurring?

---

feeling problem, etc.? In any case of uncertainty, which we believe occurrs nearly all the time, it is better for the therapist to inquire about the *how*, rather than believing that he or she really knows. How the situation constitutes a problem directly leads the therapist into the client's experience of the problem and helps define more clearly the aspect of the problem that the intervention should address. As you read the clinical examples in this chapter, note the many variations and idiosyncracies of "how" depression constitutes a problem.

Another very useful aspect of describing the nature of the complaint is pursuing information regarding when the problem *isn't* occurring and what the client is already doing that is helping the problem (de Shazer, 1985). These questions attempt to identify exceptions to the problem that may be useful to either expand in the interview process itself (see next section) or incorporate into interventions that build upon or amplify the exceptions between sessions. Questions to obtain information about the problem *not* happening are also presented in Table 4.1.

Example

Mark was a 38-year-old college student referred by an employee assistance program (EAP) for depression. Following the therapist's initial questions, Mark described himself as depressed and very sensitive to events occurring around him. He cited an example when he felt very depressed as a result of watching the evening news. The therapist pursued the nature of Mark's depression by asking him how the depression was a problem for him. Mark replied that it affected his ability to concentrate on his homework and during tests, and he added that he spent much of his time worrying about his seemingly increasing inability to concentrate. The therapist asked if there were ever times that Mark was able to concentrate and didn't worry about it as much. Mark responded that he concentrated better at school studying with his classmates. Pursuing what behaviorally constituted Mark's depression and how it was a problem revealed a problem of concentration and worry that was improved around classmates at school.

How the Problem is Being Handled

The next step is to ask what all the persons closely involved with the problem have been doing to try to handle or resolve it. Those closely involved, in addition to the client, may include family members, friends, fellow workers, professionals, and so on, depending on the circumstances of the particular case. Again, this inquiry focuses on actual behaviors, what people are doing and saying in their attempts to prevent a recurrence of the problem, or on how they deal with it when it does happen.

The therapist is attempting to determine what recursive sequence of behaviors occurs around the problem and what kinds of client and other solution attempts are maintaining the problem. A full appreciation of solution attempts is crucial from the MRI level of change, because over time it is the solutions themselves that become the problem and, therefore, must be interrupted for problem resolution to occur. The intervention is directly designed from information regarding the attempted solutions of the client and usually represents a shift in the opposite direction from the basic thrust of the unsuccessful attempted solutions.

There are at least four types of attempted solutions to be investigated: those that have failed to help the problem, those that have helped (a little bit or fleetingly), those advised by others (including previous therapists), and those that have been considered by the client, but not implemented (Heath & Atkinson, 1989). This line of inquiry can steer the therapist away from interventions that have already failed, as well as provide direction toward what may be helpful to consider. Investigating solution attempts requires patience and persistence on the part of the therapist, but it is well worth the time and effort to avoid pitfalls, as well as glean the interactional context of the problem and its solutions. In one case in which a man, Scott, had been in therapy on and off for 20 years, it took two complete sessions just to discuss what previous therapists had suggested. The information obtained proved to be very helpful in not only avoiding what had not been helpful, but also in the construction of an intervention that was appreciably different from the prior unsuccessful approaches to the problem.

Scott had been in a variety of different types of therapy including insight-oriented and behavioral, as well as group therapy for the treatment of his depression. Every technique that one could imagine, as well as every antidepressant medication available, had been utilized. All of the treatments, of course, were directed toward changing the depression. At the level of change focused on interrupting repetitively applied solution attempts, the therapist intervened by discussing the dangers of change and advocated a position that change must be fraught with disadvantages and pitfalls, or the depression would likely have been improved by the previous therapeutic attempts. The therapist continued the discussion of "dangers" (Fisch et al., 1982) by asking the client to think about it more and discuss it with his wife. Another discussion revealed a wide variety of pitfalls in getting over the depression, including returning to working outside the home and no longer being primary caregiver for his children, as well as possibly unsettling his wife's long-held role of caretaking him and "handling" the family's business/ financial affairs. From that discussion, the client concluded that he should consider either working part-time or starting a business out of his home. He also added that his wife would just have to adjust to him and deal with his not being depressed any more. Therapy proceeded in that vein and, over time, Scott began a landscaping business and dropped out of therapy.

On occasions where solutions have succeeded, or exceptions (de Shazer et al., 1986) to the problem where clients are able to handle or overcome the problem, it may be helpful to construct an intervention that incorporates and builds upon those successes. Questions regarding solution attempts are presented in Table 4.2.

It is necessary to attempt to understand the basic theme of the various efforts being made. While a client may try a variety of attempted solutions from multiple sources, they may well be variations on a central theme that is discernable, as in the case of Mark.

Mark

Investigating Mark's solutions revealed that he had tried reminding himself of his past successes in school since he had completed an undergraduate degree many years earlier. Mark also told himself how stupid he was for worrying and pressured himself severely to concentrate harder by thinking of how badly he would feel if he indeed failed. Mark seemed to try reassurance, followed by self-criticism and pressure, and attempts to force or will himself to concentrate. Others had followed a

TABLE 4.2. Questions Regarding Solution Attempts and Small Goal Formulation

What have you done about the problem?

How did these attempts work?

Have you shared this situation with others?

What did they advise or suggest?

Did it work?

Anyone else suggest anything?

Have you considered trying something else, but didn't acutally follow through with it?

What, when it happens, will you see as a first sign that a significant, although small, change has occurred?

What will be an indication that things are beginning to turn toward problem improvement?

(If something is already happening) What will be the next sign?

If this problem was rated on a scale of 1–10, with 10 being no problem at all, and 1 being as bad as it gets, where are you now? What would the next higher number look like?

If you went to sleep tonight and a miracle occurred and cured this probelm, what would be the first thing you would notice different when you first opened your eyes?

How will you know that you don't have to come here anymore? What will be different?

How will you know when he or she has a better attitude, has improved self-esteem, etc.?

What will you be doing differently when this (symptom) is less of a current problem in your life?

What will you be doing differently with your time?

What useful things will you be in the habit of saying to yourself?

What will you be thinking about (doing) instead of thinking about the (problem)?

What do you think that (significant other, referring agency, probation officer, etc.) would say is the first sign that things are getting better?

What do you think he or she will notice first?

What do you think your (significant other) will begin to notice about you as this is less of a problem?

What would convince (significant other or other agency invested in the client receiving and responding to treatment) that you need to come here less often (or not at all)?

similar theme of solution attempts by suggesting that he not worry, that he would do fine, and finally that he should seek help. Mark's troubles with concentration and worry occurred within an interactional cycle consisting of a variety of efforts to reassure and browbeat himself to concentrate, which decreased his ability to concentrate, which led to more worrying and more reassurance from others and self-criticism, etc.

Client's Minimal Goals

Inquiry about the client's minimal goals of treatment may be the most difficult aspect for the therapist about the first interview. Some people do not think in terms of goals and specific outcome criteria, so it is often much easier to obtain a general or abstract formulation of the goals, rather than one that will signify that the problem is resolving and the therapeutic process is working. Despite the inherent difficulties for the therapist with some clients in certain instances, it is important to pursue a collaborative definition of a goal that will allow everyone involved in the problematic situation to know that therapy is moving in the right direction. With respectful perseverance, a therapist can elicit a pertinent response that serves as an outcome criterion. Even if the questions regarding specific goals bear no fruit, the pursuit itself serves an important function. At the least, the therapist will likely be perceived as interested in change, and therapy as being about change (Fisch et al., 1982). We will elaborate on this aspect of goal formulation later in the chapter.

Think Small

It is most helpful to encourage the client to think small. Because a basic assumption is that a small change leads to additional changes, the logical place to start is with a first small step. If one person changes, the relationship also changes. If one family member changes, other family members also change. A change in one aspect of an individual's life often leads to changes in other areas as well.

The wonderful thing about getting people to think small is that the small goal often represents the larger problem to the client. Attainment of the small goal becomes symbolic of resolving the entire problem. It doesn't matter how small the goal may seem, the client's minimal goal can be connected to and representative of a far greater goal. The therapeutic task, then, is to achieve small goals that ultimately are more meaningful to the client than first glance might indicate.

For example, Edward, a 47-year-old salesman, presented his problem as depression and an inability to follow through with his work responsibilities. When asked what an indication would be if things were on the right track, Edward replied that he would make his schedule on Mondays and then follow through with his appointments the rest of the week. The therapist responded that perhaps that goal was a good one but maybe a little big and asked what would be the first indication that things were beginning to turn in the right direction. Edward thought for a while and replied that he would be flossing his teeth before he went to bed. Flossing his teeth came to represent not being depressed to Edward. Do not underestimate the power of thinking small. Questions related to small goal formulation are also presented in Table 4.2.

If this line of questioning reveals nothing specific, then you have learned an important aspect of the client's meaning system and how he or she organizes his or her perception and experience. You have learned that the client experiences the world in a way that does not break down linguistically into discrete and concrete chunks.

Mark

Recall Mark and his worrying and concentration problem. Pursuit of Mark's minimal goal resulted in Mark formulating the goal of being able to study for one hour at home without worrying or losing concentration for more than a few minutes. From the level of change that views strategy as interrupting the behavioral interaction that constitutes the problem cycle, the following information was elicited from the interview format permitting an interactive description of the problem process.

Nature of the Problem

> *Who*: Mark
> *What*: Depression; feeling depressed
> *To whom*: Mark
> *How*: Inability to concentrate; worrying about same
> *Exceptions*: When studying with classmates

Client's Solutions Attempts

> 1. Don't worry
> 2. This is stupid
> 3. I've done this before
> 4. Other's solutions similar in theme

Client's Minimal Goals

Able to study for 1 hour without worrying or losing concentration. Attempting to interrupt the problem cycle by asking Mark to do something different than his stated solution attempts, the therapist designed an intervention based in Mark's noted exception to the problem. Mark was asked to observe the differences between when he was able to concentrate at school with his classmates and when he was at home and didn't concentrate as well, and to pay particular attention to how he was able to overcome his worry and focus his concentration (de Shazer, 1985).

REVISING ITS MEANING

To this point, based in the level of change that seeks to interrupt the problem cycle, the interview format had elicited the particulars of the client's everyday life experience, highlighting the specific aspects that the client finds problematic, the client's unsuccessful solutions, and a mutually formulated, minimal goal. Yet the interview entails far more than the passive absorption of interactive information for the design of a problem-process interrupting intervention. By the phrasing of questions, responses to client's comments and questions, and guiding the therapeutic conversation itself, the therapist is simultaneously constructing opportunities for client change.

Through the interview itself, the therapist attempts to construct a frame surrounding the client's presenting problem that allows for problem resolution to occur. From the level of change that views strategy as promoting meaning revision through the conversational recreation of the client's experience, the interview may revise the client's frame of reference or definition of the problem. Meanings ascribed to problem situations are open to revision when clients tell their stories to the therapist.

An interview not only elicits a description of the problem and its meaning to the client, but also is an inherently interventive process of coevolving the client's formulation of those meanings. The therapist and the client are cocreating what the client experiences as a problem as the client unfolds the content of the problem story. Every client story presents the opportunity for saying the heretofore never said, and the cogeneration of new perceptions and meanings. From the revision of meaning level of change, the interview format is an ongoing quest for opportunities to evolve new meanings (Anderson & Goolishian, 1988).

Telling the Story

Therapy begins by inviting clients to tell their stories, "What brings you here today?" In the course of telling their stories, clients provide their informal theory regarding the problem and give the therapist an idea of their orientations toward life, their goals and ambitions, and the pressures and events surrounding their complaints. In short, clients unfold the content of their lives, their meaning system, which organizes their perceptions and experiences. The problem story represents a therapeutic entry point in the client's life and is, at the point of entry, an opportunity to revise the meanings in the story that are distressing to the client.

The therapist respectfully and patiently listens to the story. Although it may seem counterproductive, the client should have complete freedom to tell the whole story without interruption by the therapist. The therapist is sensitive to openings for his or her comments, but does not distract clients from telling the stories that brought them to therapy. Some clients may give 30-second descriptions and look to the therapist for immediate questions, while others may have been sitting on their stories for a long time and need to share lengthy narratives. In any event, as we have emphasized, the therapist must be sensitive to what appears to be the client's needs in the interview, and respond accordingly. In addition to providing the therapist with clients' content description of their meaning systems, the client's initial narrative is also a potentially powerful validating experience. We will elaborate on the validation component in the next section. For now, our interest is in constructing frames that promote change as well as in evolving new meanings via the interview format.

Nature of the Problem: Revisited

The pursuit of an interactional description of the presenting problem is itself part of a process that constructs a frame around the problem that enables opportunities for change. Just getting the client to present the situation in concrete terms may be a therapeutic accomplishment because often a client's abstract descriptions of problematic situations offer little possibility for change and make it difficult to identify possible solutions (Coyne, 1986). For example, depression is a general and vague (although valid) problem description that offers little direction for corrective action. Asking *what* the person is depressed about or *how* the depression is a problem begins the co-construction of a frame of reference about the problem that permits the problem to be changed or improved. Recall Mark the student and Edward the salesman. Both problem descriptions were lifted out of the general frame of depression and placed in the idiosyncratically formed frames of trouble concentrating and not following through, respectively. Depression offers limited options for change, while problems of concentration and follow through permit a more directly changeable frame of the problem. The pursuit of specificity, then, also helps define the problem in such a way that allows for more solution options.

Research addressing how people specify their actions suggests that when led to think about the details of their actions and situations, they are more likely to redefine or ascribe new or revised meaning to their situations (Wegner, Vallocher, Macomber, Wood, & Arps, 1984). Similarly, being required through therapist questions to attend painstakingly to the details of their situations may promote opportunities for clients to ascribe different meanings to their situations (Coyne, 1986). The pursuit of specificity allows for distinctions to be drawn and observations to be made that were previously undrawn and unmade. Attention to detailed aspects of the client's description enhances the human tendency to attribute meaning to experience and creates opportunities for coevolution of new meanings.

Abstractions not only limit remedial actions, but also prevent people from considering the full implications of their circumstances. Linda, a 28-year-old woman, described her problem as "clinical depression," as diagnosed by her well-meaning pastor. The therapist asked the client what she was depressed about, and the client responded by describing a recent move and a variety of subsequent losses, as well as a firm dislike for the climate of the new city. The therapist pursued the "what" question and asked if there was anything else about the move in addition to the losses and bad climate that was depressing to her. The client thought for a while, and responded that the new city was much like her hometown, which brought up several traumatic memories from her childhood. Linda added that the move perhaps reminded her of a series of sexual encounters she had experienced as a child. Pursuit of the details associated with the "what" of her depression resulted in the implication that the move was more significant than she had previously considered.

Creating Opportunities Through Conversation

The first interview is a therapist-guided storytelling experience that promotes meaning revision through the unfolding of conversation. The therapeutic conversation is a collaborative search and exploration through discussion, and coauthorship of ideas and meanings that create an ever-present opportunity for clients to reexperience their problem situations (Anderson & Goolishian, 1988). The first interview (and therapy in general) is a continual process of unfolding, expanding, revising, and creating meaning.

Through the detailed pursuit of the presenting problem, the client's attempted solutions, and minimal therapy goals, the content of the problem is thoroughly explored, and other descriptions, connections, implications, and distinctions can emerge. The client's content focus defines the nature of the therapist's questions. The therapist works within the client's informal content focus and respectfully and slowly adds to it or questions it. The therapist works to learn and converse in the client's language and attempts to impose as little content as possible to the client's presentation. Conversing in the client's language is respectful and conveys understanding, and prevents the imposition of different connotations not intended by the client. The therapist pays attention to the words the client uses because they represent the client's view of his or her life. The therapist also listens for the client's style of presenting the problem in terms of whether it is action oriented, thinking oriented, and/or feeling oriented. Attention to the client's style enables a more client-specific empathic response by the therapist, and provides direction regarding between-session assignments.

Therapist questions elicit information and construct a frame of reference for psychotherapy itself. The questions create a changeable problem definition and facilitate the cogeneration of different meanings. Each question in the interview format offers an opportunity for meaning revision. Each question may unfold the client's story in such a way as to open a therapeutic path to changing the presenting problem. Sometimes, the questions lead to revisions in meaning that render the rest of the interview unnecessary or irrelevant. Other times, a meaning may evolve, and an opportunity may be pursued, but the path does not lead to problem improvement. In such instances, the therapist returns to the interview format and continues to pursue a detailed description of the presenting problem.

The interview format constructs opportunities for change and creates a frame that promotes change. Recall Linda, the 28-year-old woman presenting with clinical depression. Further exploration of the "what" question resulted in the client's connecting her recent move and what she was depressed about to traumatic sexual experiences from childhood. The pursuit of details about her depression led to an unfolding of a connection that was previously unsaid by the client. Therapist questions are intended to create a context for the heretofore unstated, promoting the evolution of new meanings and opening pathways to problem resolution. With the client's permission, the therapist pursued the client-presented content of her sexual encounters in childhood. It is important to note that the connection between the depression and the childhood sexual experiences was made by the client, and it was therefore her informal theory of her depression that the therapist pursued. The therapist did not impose any formal content.

Pursuing the path introduced by the client's connection led to the client's description of an ongoing series of sexually abusive incidents involving the client at ages 8–10 and her 15–17-year-old female cousin. The client had described the incidents to her pastor several years before, and he suggested to her that it sounded like "playing doctor." The therapist respectfully added to the story that playing doctor involved the curious looking and touching of same-aged peers and not the power-disparate abuse of a child by an adolescent seeking sexual gratification at the child's expense. The client's feelings of guilt and shame dissipated as she recreated her experiences through the lens of abuse, rather than playing doctor. The "what" question enabled a new connection between her depression and her sexual abuse. The therapist took the opportunity presented by the client and proceeded down the path of revising the client's meaning about sexual abuse. The rest of the interview format became irrelevant because the emergent opportunity took precedence.

The case of Mark illustrates how the first interview constructs a frame that promotes change, lifting the problem out of a difficult-to-change depression frame and placing it in an easier-to-change concentration problem frame. The case of Linda illustrates how the first interview constructs opportunities for change by unfolding the client's content- rich description of the presenting problem.

Attempted Solutions and Client Minimal Goals: Revisited

The interview questions are a vehicle to enable a fluid conversation in which the focus is in the direction of evolving new meanings. The questions are designed to impose minimal therapist content and to allow maximum space for the client to find new connections, distinctions, and meanings. The questions are not designed to influence *particular* meanings or to distinguish between health and pathology or any other formal theory content-based reality.

The kinds of questions a therapist asks and the data that are extracted from the interview are powerful determinants in creating a reality that either promotes change or discourages it. If therapists ask about sleep, appetite, and sex habits, many endogenous depressions will be constructed, which will be treated with antidepressants, which will lead to further investigation of the client's sleep, appetite, and sex habits (Rosenbaum, 1990).

Be cautious about the frame of reference you construct around the problem. Do not impose a theoretical content that defines the problem as difficult to change or that lifts the problem out of the client's frame of reference. Stay within the client's frame and add to it as it unfolds over time through the therapeutic conversation. The perils of a therapist-imposed frame are illustrated in the following case.

Don

Don, a 49-year-old recently separated man, was referred for depression growing out of his wife Cindy's decision to leave the marriage of 5 years. The referral source had indicated that he had great concerns for Don's lethality should Cindy decide to follow through with her decision. Don confirmed that he did indeed consider suicide a possibility if his wife did not return; he had a .38-caliber revolver in his home. The matter-of-fact quality to this assertion was convincing. Prior to the end of the first session, the therapist secured a no-suicide contract with Don, wherein he committed himself to contact the therapist prior to any attempt on his life.

The therapist saw Don weekly thereafter, during which time Cindy continued on course to dissolve the marriage, giving Don a relatively consistent message that the marriage was over as far as she was concerned. Don maintained that he was sure he could get Cindy back if only he could make her see how miserable he was without her. Hence, his strategy essentially consisted of efforts to woo her from a position of neediness and dependency. At one point early in the work, Cindy telephoned in a panicky voice to relate that she felt Don was very suicidal, and had in fact threatened her with his suicide should she decide to leave him.

Don's initial goal for therapy was to learn how to get Cindy back. His view had been that if he could get her back, he would no longer be depressed and would, in fact, be fine. The therapist's concerns with his lethality, in spite of Don's comments that as long as there existed a chance for reunification, he had no imminent plans to kill himself, became paramount in the work. The therapist spent each session exploring with him the state of his mood, which was virtually always depressed, and the level of suicidal ideation he carried. His answer was always the same: Fears about his lethality could not be quelled in spite of Don's assurances. The therapy went nowhere. As the therapist worked a suicide prevention agenda, Don grew frustrated that therapy was not helping him get his wife back. The singular focus on Don's "suicidal alternative" and clinical efforts to avoid his selecting this option had in effect arrested progress toward achieving his goal of getting his wife back.

Soon thereafter, the treatment team converged, and another therapist interviewed Don to get a restatement of Don's view and goals for therapy. He admitted to feeling depressed and at times fleetingly suicidal, but denied any current intent. Don acknowledged that he possessed a gun, and had no plan to remove it from his home. He reassured the interviewing therapist that he didn't plan on using the gun on himself unless he failed to get Cindy back. Then, Don said, it might be a different story.

The therapist asked Don how long he was willing to hold out like this, how long he was willing to wait for Cindy to make up her mind. Don replied he didn't think he could last more than 2 more years! The therapist had been living with the belief that each session with Don might be the last! The team, after consultation with the interviewing therapist, suggested to Don that the best shot he had at getting Cindy back was to pull himself together and prove to her that he was not as needy and dependent as she thought him to be, and that he might want to consider pulling himself together so he could preserve his stamina for a 2-year marital siege. Don saw some merit to these suggestions, recognizing that one of Cindy's complaints about him was that he depended on her too much.

Thereafter, the therapy with Don progressed well, with the goal being to help him stabilize his mood and carry on with life, not as a means of letting go of Cindy, but as a possible way of getting her back. This Don worked toward with a great amount of success. During the course of developing his new independence, Don discovered that he didn't need Cindy nearly as much as he had originally thought. When, 3 months later, she filed for divorce, he was upset and very tearful at the prospect of losing her, but had decided that living would be the best revenge. The therapist's active collaboration in defining the problem as Don's suicidal ideation and the ongoing focus on that problem led to a continual confirmation of the therapist's fears and expectations.

Attempted Solutions

Pursuing the client's attempted solutions yields an interactive description of the problem and prevents the therapeutic pitfall of suggesting something that the client has already tried without success. Such a pursuit also offers an opportunity for the exploration of solutions that have worked previously, ones that are currently helping, or ones that the client may be considering. The therapist may view any of the previous solution attempts as a noteworthy exception to the problem in that the solutions may represent times when the client is already experiencing success. Such successes indicate therapeutic opportunities that the therapist may act upon to expand with a series of questions. Questions building upon small exceptions or successful solutions can open a therapeutic path that results in the cogeneration of different meanings and/or a new solution to the problem. Again, such openings may render the rest of the interview format unnecessary, or may ultimately lead to a dead end.

Margaret, a 36-year-old single parent presented herself as depressed about her 17-year-old's pot smoking. Her son, Brent, refused to attend sessions. Investigating Margaret's solution attempts revealed that she had tried a variety of things, including lectures, groundings, and education at a chemical dependency unit, but none of her attempts had influenced her son's regular pot use. The therapist asked if Margaret was considering any other solutions, but had not yet implemented them. Margaret replied that she was thinking of subjecting Brent to a urine test and requiring clean urine before allowing him to participate in his favorite summer pastime of sailing, which was an expensive hobby that Mom helped to fund. The therapist asked the client how she came to that solution and other questions designed to unfold her perspective and expand her resolve to address Brent's pot abuse. Such empowering questions enable the client to draw upon previous knowledge, and often encourage clients to experience a sense of self-efficacy. Margaret responded by saying that she had been pushed around for too long by Brent and made to feel guilty about initiating the breakup of her marriage. She knew now that feeling guilty about her affair and broken marriage just distracted her from doing what needed to be done. The therapist added that Margaret might consider application of her solution right away to Brent's driving privileges.

The questions about solutions constructed an opportunity surrounding Margaret's resolve to address Brent's pot smoking. The path that opened led to an unfolding of self-empowering meanings by the client and a clear solution to her problem. The client's content (urine check) provided the content of the solution, not the therapist's theoretical orientation.

Minimal Goals

Asking clients about their minimal goals for therapy provides the therapist with specific outcome criteria upon which to determine progress and gives clients the message that the therapist is interested in change. Asking questions regarding goals also helps construct a frame that promotes change and creates opportunities for meaning revision. Recall Edward and how goal questions helped construct a reality for change. Edward responded to the goal question with the surprising answer that flossing his teeth would represent a sign that his problem, first described as depression, would be better. Achievement of the goal of flossing teeth was seen as a far easier therapeutic task than curing Edward's depression. When Edward did achieve teeth flossing, he also achieved a significant improvement in his follow-through on the job. He also no longer felt depressed.

Bob, a single 45-year-old, presented with a long description of his "chronic depression." Bob had been in insight-oriented therapy for 2 years previously, but decided to try someone new at his ex-lover's insistence. Unfolding the content of Bob's story revealed Bob to be struggling with the loss of a relationship and his rebellious adolescent son. The therapist asked Bob how he would know when he didn't have to come back for therapy any more. Bob was somewhat puzzled, and the therapist repeated the question. Bob commented that he had never been asked that question before by a therapist and added that he thought therapy was an ongoing thing. The therapist replied that some therapists work that way and that was okay, but that he liked to know what he and Bob would be working toward, even in a long-term, slow fashion.

Bob said that he would know that therapy was over when he started living his life and began doing things to make himself feel better. He added that he understood what the therapist was driving at—that he (Bob) was in charge of his life and that he would have to make the changes if he were ever to get over his depression. The therapist asked what changes Bob was referring to, and Bob answered that he would take flying lessons and stop bailing his son out of trouble. The therapist inquired about what the first step toward those changes would be. Bob responded that he would make an appointment with a flight instructor. Bob returned for session two and announced that he had had his first lesson and that he was ready to leave therapy and fly solo.

The question about how Bob would know when therapy was finished created an opportunity for a revision in Bob's meanings about therapy itself and his depression. The pursuit of the goal seemed to allow Bob to make distinctions and draw conclusions that were previously unsaid and unmade. The therapist followed the opportunity presented by the client and proceeded to continue asking the goals questions and expanding and unfolding Bob's newly ascribed meanings. The therapist responded to the new content Bob added about making changes in his life by asking questions that required more articulation by Bob regarding what the changes would be. Bob connected his depression to the way he was living his life, a heretofore unspoken connection that was only empowered further by additional questions. Each therapist question, including those that pursue details concerning the client's minimal goals, contain the possibility for opening a pathway that leads to meaning revision. The initial interview is an ongoing quest for these meaning revising opportunities.

VALIDATING THE CLIENT'S EXPERIENCE

To this point, the initial interview has been discussed in terms of eliciting an interactional description to enable an interruption of the problem process and as a method of constructing change opportunities via the conversational unfolding and exploring of the client's content-rich meaning system. Yet, once again, the interview involves far more than eliciting information or the quest for meaning revision opportunities. The first interview is the principle medium through which the therapist defines the nature of the therapist–client relationship as one that is empathic, respectful, and genuine as perceived by the client. The relationship is also defined as one in which an inherent therapeutic goal is to validate the client's experience of the world and replace the invalidation that sometimes accompanies clients to therapy.

Initial impressions are very important. Recall that early indicators of the therapeutic alliance from the first three sessions are powerful predictors of positive outcome. This underscores the paramount importance of therapist sensitivity to the client's perception of the common factors as well as the client's views regarding the tasks and goals of therapy.

Setting a common factors context and addressing the goal of validation begins simply by merely listening and allowing the client to tell his or her story. Beyond permitting the client to unfold the content related to his or her problem, the therapist is sensitive to openings that can serve as validation. The telling of the story itself can provide validation as the following fable implies.

> When the great Rabbi Israel Baal Shem-Tov saw misfortune threatening the Jews, it was his custom to go into a certain part of the forest to meditate. There he would light a fire, say a special prayer, and the miracle would be accomplished and the misfortune averted.
>
> Later, when his disciple, the celebrated Magid of Mezritch, had occasion, for the same reason, to intercede with heaven, he would go to the same place in the forest and say: "Master of the Universe, listen! I do not know how to light the fire, but I am still able to say the prayer." And again the miracle would be accomplished.
>
> Still later, Rabbi Moshe-Leib of Sasov, in order to save his people once more, went to the forest and said: "I do not know how to light the fire, I do not know the prayer, but I know the place and this must by sufficient." It was sufficient and the miracle was accomplished.
>
> Then it fell to Rabbi Israel of Rizhyn to overcome misfortune. Sitting in his armchair, his head in his hands, he spoke to God: "I am unable to light the fire and I do not know the prayer; I cannot even find the place in the forest. All I can do is to tell the story, and this must be sufficient." And it was sufficient. God made man because he loves stories. (Wiesel, 1966, pp. i-iv)

Perhaps another meaning of this fable is that the validation that occurs in telling the story is itself curative and potentially powerful in resolving client concerns.

Validating the client's experience begins with the therapist genuinely holding the attitude that clients are doing the best they can under the circumstances and that their presentations make sense, given what is happening in their lives (Coyne, 1986)—simple concept, but very difficult to enact. If the therapist cannot appreciate that a client's presentation makes sense, it is likely that the therapist has not allowed enough of the client's story to unfold and needs to focus attention toward expanding and exploring the context of the problem.

The next consideration is therapeutic sensitivity to openings for validation. Clients present with great variability. Clients may unfold their stories in lengthy narratives and give little space for a therapist's verbal input. The therapist does not interfere with the story because, as alluded to earlier, the telling of the story is itself a powerful validation when told to an empathic and accepting listener. Clients hear their own voices telling of their experiences and find validation in doing so (Parry, 1991).

At other times, clients leave space for therapist responses, which can present openings for therapeutic validation. Recall that validation occurs when the client's thoughts, feelings, and behaviors are accepted, believed, and considered completely understandable given the client's subjective experience of the world. Such an opening occurred quickly with Mark, the 38-year-old student who initially presented that he was very sensitive to events around him and could become easily depressed as a result of watching the evening news. After a pause, the therapist commented that watching the death and destruction of the Gulf War and contemplating the impact on the involved individuals and families was indeed quite depressing. In and of itself, that is not all that significant, but such statements set the context of psychotherapy toward validating the client's experience. Mark agreed with the therapist and went on to further explain his concerns.

As Mark discussed his problems with concentration and worrying, and what others had suggested to him (don't worry, reassurance), his narrative was often punctuated with how stupid the whole problem was, given his past successes. Further conversation revealed that Mark had returned to college to finally pursue a career that was very important to him. His previous college experience was viewed by Mark as boring and unmeaningful because it led to a series of unsatisfactory employments. This time, however, meant everything: He was no longer a kid resting on potential, and if he didn't succeed at school this time, it essentially meant he was a failure. Therefore, not concentrating represented a far greater life tragedy than merely not doing well on a test or in a class. Not concentrating and poor performance in school was Mark's whole life on the line. Imagine the invalidation of "don't worry" and reassurance. It was like telling a person driving off of a cliff to not worry about the fall.

The therapist said to Mark in many ways, "No wonder you are worrying and having trouble concentrating, this is not just a class, it's your career and your life. It is all of your self-worth rolled up into one do or die experience." With encouragement by the therapist's comments, Mark found validation of his experience of distress that replaced the invalidation of other (don't worry) and his own invalidations (this is stupid). Mark no longer experienced the incongruence between what he felt as extremely distressing and what others described as trivial.

Validation versus Normalization

Validation is very different than what some have called normalization. Normalization is used as a way to offer commonplace explanations and to shrug off clients' concerns as not newsworthy (O'Hanlon & Weiner-Davis, 1989). O'Hanlon and Weiner-Davis (1989) liken normalization to how physicians reassure their patients less by what they say than what they don't seem to regard as even worth remarking upon. Although such normalizations may help clients who fear being crazy or believe that they are alone in experiencing problems, such an approach may minimize clients' concerns and trivialize their experience. Mark's distress may have been further invalidated by normalizing comments such as "naturally," "of course," "that sounds familiar," or "so what else is new?" (O'Hanlon & Weiner-Davis, 1989). Validation requires that therapist comments *highlight* the importance of the client's experience and its utter *justification* given the context of their lives.

Validation of the client's subjective experience of the world is a powerful enhancer of common factors. How better for the therapist to convey empathy, respect, and genuineness than to listen to the client, understand the importance of the his or her concern, and communicate how completely justifiable the client's thoughts, feelings, and behaviors are, given their circumstances. Validation requires acceptance of the client's meaning system at face value. This sometimes requires the therapist to accept and respect the validity of unusual ideas and behaviors. Such a validation of even bizarre meaning systems opens the door for the therapist and the client to generate new meanings. Validation of the existing frame of reference allows flexibility of that frame of reference. Recall Joe from Chapter 3 and the therapist's acceptance of a "delusional" meaning system. Validating that frame of reference enabled a shift in Joe's meaning system that no longer included delusional thinking.

Sometimes clients offer special challenges to therapists regarding validation, and certain situations demand great patience by the therapist. But it is worth it when it results in replacing an invalidating experience brought by the client with a validating one that opens possibilities for rapid change.

Validation: Special Challenges

Consider Richard, a 25-year-old systems analyst, referred by his company doctor because of Richard's obvious distress and preoccupation on the job. Richard looked quite agitated and immediately greeted his therapist in the waiting room with a demanding, "What are you going to do for me?" The therapist answered by showing him to his office, and Richard repeated his question. Richard seemed quite hostile, and the therapist was uncomfortable. The therapist, however, believed that if he could get Richard to tell his story, it would all make sense, hostility, agitation, and all.

The therapist replied that he didn't know if he could help and could Richard please tell him what brought him to see him. Richard told his story.

Richard began suspecting his wife of having an affair after he discovered unidentified footprints in the snow. Other bits of evidence (telephone hang-ups, staying out later than expected) resulted in Richard beginning to check the bed sheets for signs of semen, which would provide ironclad evidence of her unfaithfulness (given there was no recent sex with him). Throughout Richard's growing mistrust, his wife emphatically denied the affair, told him he was crazy, and filed for divorce. Richard continued checking the bedsheets until he found stains. He took the sheet to a laboratory, which confirmed the presence of semen. His wife still denied his accusations and insisted the semen was his. His wife began telling friends and family, including their own children, that Richard was paranoid and sick.

Apologizing for his apparent distress and paranoia, Richard told the therapist that he was obtaining a DNA profile of the semen to see if it matched his own DNA profile. Richard nervously asked the therapist if he believed him. The therapist responded that he, indeed, believed him and thought he had good reason to suspect his wife.

Explicit to the nature of the therapeutic relationship is the therapist's validation and acceptance of the client's subjective experience of the world. Validation and acceptance do not require agreement with the therapist's personal opinions, and it is not the therapist's job to point out the differences when they occur.

After Richard told the therapist about the DNA test, Richard also asked the therapist if he thought he was crazy for spending $1200. The therapist replied that peace of mind is cheap at any price. The therapist was moved by Richard's tearful reply of "thank you." It seemed that the company doctor had told him that he was imagining things, and the DNA test was a waste of money.

By allowing Richard to tell his story and not getting sidetracked by Richard's initial presentation or by attributions of pathology, the therapist was permitted to make sense of Richard's hostility and agitation. No wonder he was hostile, given that others had essentially told him he was crazy and wasting his family's money. In the context of the therapeutic relationship, Richard found validation of his concerns to replace the invalidation of his experiences that others' descriptions of them implied. The therapist and Richard collaborated on a plan for Richard to deal with his suspicions, and he ultimately divorced his wife. The validation seemed to enable Richard to expand his frame of reference to include proactive behaviors concerning his job, children, and decision to divorce.

Recall Linda, the sexually abused woman who believed that her sexual experiences constituted playing doctor. Playing doctor, the description that another helper ascribed to her experience, was an invalidating description. Playing doctor implied that nothing of any consequence really happened, yet the client felt extremely guilty and distressed about the experiences. So not only did she feel deeply troubled by the experiences, she also had to contend with a description of her experiences that implied she shouldn't feel distressed. The telling of the story allowed for Linda's distress to be validated by the term *sexual abuse*, which replaced the invalidation that playing doctor implied.

Validation is really empathy to its logical extension. Empathy is accepting and attempting to understand and work within the expressed meaning system of the client. Empathy is essentially accepting the client's frame of reference as the theoretical orientation that guides therapy. Validation requires not only acceptance of the meaning system, but also an outright verbal justification of the client's meaning system by the therapist. We believe that a therapist's attitude that promotes validation enhances common factors and sets the context for client change. If nothing else occurs except validation in the initial interview, then the interview is a resounding success. Sometimes, validation is all that is required to enable clients to resolve their difficulties.

INTERVIEWING COUPLES AND FAMILIES: ADDITIONAL CONSIDERATIONS

Perhaps solely by virtue of bringing an additional person or persons into the therapeutic context, marital and family therapy offers the therapist special challenges as well as multiple opportunities for change. The dramatic intensity with which couples and families may present (e.g., an affair or child involved with drugs), the occasional polarization of viewpoints, and the difficulty inherent in validating each person's perspective without disconfirming the others' can offer a humbling experience to the most seasoned of therapists.

In order to begin the interview process and the quest for change opportunities described in this chapter, it is necessary first to decide who will be interviewed. Because any or all persons who are attempting to solve the problem can impact the problem cycle by doing something different, there are no rigid guidelines that govern who must be seen. For example, it is possible for a parent with a child problem or a spouse with a marital problem to effect change in the problem cycle without bringing the child or spouse to therapy. However, if more than one person involved in the problematic interaction is interested in resolving the problem, then possible intervention alternatives are multiplied, as are entry points into the problem cycle.

As in all other decision points concerning treatment, it is best to follow the client's view of how treatment should unfold. If there is an opportunity to discuss this issue prior to the first session, clients are generally asked to include individuals in treatment that they believe to be relevant to solving the problem. If clients describe the problem as marital or familial, then clients may be encouraged to invite their spouses and other family members to therapy. Similar to other aspects of our approach, clients are met on their own terms, and the therapist will at least begin with whomever chooses to attend, and will continue with that focus as long as it appears to be influencing the attainment of the client's goals.

While offering special challenges, marital and family therapy enables a variety of options regarding entry points in the couple or family's problematic experiences. To maximize opportunities, it is helpful to set the context for marital and family therapy by interviewing the couple or family together *and* separately. With families, this generally entails interviewing the child or adolescent separate from the parents. Usually, unless a client requests separate interviews at the onset, the interview begins with the couple or family together and then proceeds to separate interviews.

The interview starts by obtaining an initial problem statement from each individual. If there appears to be agreement regarding what the problem is, or there is disagreement, but an open flow of ideas, the therapist may continue conversation regarding a description of the problem with all individuals present. However, if there is immediate disagreement that shuts down one individual, or there appears to be tension that is preventing an exchange of views, then it is better to split the couple or family and proceed with separate interviews.

Couples and families usually respond favorably and seem to understand the utility of separate interviews. The therapist simply explains that he or she would like to see each person separately (or split the generations) and asks which one prefers to go first. This often allows the person(s) most distressed to gain "airtime" with the therapist immediately.

Advantages of Separate Interviews

Seeing members of a couple or family separately, in addition to as a unit, has several advantages. Separate interviews allow the therapist access to an unedited and uncensored description of each individual's perspective of the problem that led to therapy. Each individual's meaning system, therefore, is unfolded, accepted, and enlisted in service of the couple or family's goals for therapy. The therapist learns each person's views on what or who the problem is, and how each individual thinks it should be addressed. Separate interviews affords the therapist the opportunity to discover *who* is most interested in changing *what* problem and who may not even consider there to be a problem at all. The MRI calls this process finding out who the "customer" for change is. At the very least, the

therapist determines who may be readily engaged in the change process
and who may not be so readily involved or perhaps even interested.

Example

Wayne and LoNita jointly presented the problem as LoNita's depression.
Wayne believed the problem to be hormonally based and because the
children had all left home. LoNita stated that since the children had left,
her life lacked a purpose and she felt useless. Separate interviews revealed
a somewhat different picture. LoNita, in her separate interview, did not
mention her lack of meaning, but rather focused on Wayne's authoritarian parental style and how he had alienated their children. LoNita
described her depression as a problem with Wayne's mistreatment of the
children. Wayne, on the other hand, described the problem as LoNita's
overattention to the children and her lack of attention to him. An initial
presentation of depression ultimately yielded to two related, yet very
different descriptions of who and what the problems actually were.

Seeing couples and families separately also enables the therapist to
validate each person's perspective without concern for alienating the
other person(s). It is almost a given that couples in distress will have
differing perspectives about their problems and that children/adolescents
will have opposing views to their parent's about the presenting concerns.
Such differences are not obstacles, but rather are the vehicles through
which opportunities for change arise. Opportunity for change is enabled
by validating each person's subjective experience of the problem. This
does not require the therapist to ingenuinely represent him- or herself as
agreeing with opposite viewpoints. Rather, validation requires the
therapist to accept and legitimize genuinely those viewpoints as justifiable
given the individual's contextual vantage point.

Example

As the separate conversations unfolded with LoNita and Wayne, their
differing perspectives became apparent. The therapist validated both
LoNita's and Wayne's meaning system about LoNita's depression without
risking alienation of the other person. It was easy for the therapist to
validate LoNita's subjective experience of the problem, given her story of
how Wayne mistreated the children with his authoritarian demands. It
was similarly easy for the therapist to validate Wayne's experience of
feeling lonely and unattended to, given his descriptions of LoNita's
continual involvement in the children's lives.

Finally, separate interviews permit additional interventive possibilities given that each person's experience of the presenting problem is
addressed and each person's desires or goals are negotiated. Just as it is a

given that each individual will likely have different perspectives of the problem, it is probable that different goals for treatment will also emerge from separate interviews. While couples and families may share a goal of improving the presenting problem, how success is defined will likely be expressed idiosyncratically. The therapeutic task is to address each person's definition in such a way that success is a shared experience. Separate interviews, then, allow the therapist to intervene directly in the aspect of the problem that is most important for each individual.

Example

While both LoNita and Wayne desired a reduction of LoNita's depression, each defined success in a significantly different manner. LoNita defined success as occurring when one of their children could visit without Wayne criticizing him or her, or demanding explanations for past indiscretions. Wayne defined success as more affection from LoNita. The separate interviews allowed for access to how the experience of LoNita's depression constituted a problem and how each would indicate that improvement had occurred. Intervention, therefore, could be designed to address directly the aspect of the problem that was most important for Wayne *and* LoNita.

After the separate interviews, the couple or family is reunited, and the therapist may share any impressions or suggestions that may have arisen from the interview process. It is explained that each session will likely contain both individual and together components. Please bear in mind that the interview format is not a rigid one, and client or family needs always takes precedence. If a couple expresses a desire to sit together and hash things out with a therapist facilitator, then that desire is accepted. If a family requests sessions to help them communicate more effectively, and that means to them that all family members are present all the time, then that request is honored. The therapist should pursue the client's or family's wishes until it is clear that the desired goals are not being reached, or unless it is clear that such a format is untenable (e.g., a husband who requests the therapist to convince his wife to stay in the marriage).

Interviewing couples and families separately, as well as together, enables three sets of opportunities to promote the conditions for meaningful change (Duncan, in press). The marital or familial problems may be altered by each individual of the couple, or by the child/ adolescent or his or her parents; change may occur through any person experiencing a meaning revision or initiating a change in the problematic patterns of interaction (Duncan & Rock, 1991). In addition, intervention can encourage the couple or family also to act in concert to address a particular area of concern.

Eric, Terry, and Michelle

Eric, Terry, and their 14-year-old daughter, Michelle, were referred by the school counselor for a second opinion. The therapist began the interview with the family together and asked what brought them to see him.

Eric and Terry jointly responded with a brief description of how Michelle had been distressed of late and had brought up, on several occasions, that she intended to kill herself. They added that they went to their health maintenance organization (HMO), which offered a recommendation with which they did not agree, so they decided to seek a second opinion. Michelle stared at the floor and responded to the therapist's initial question by looking up and pointing at her parents. An overall tension seemed to characterize the interview at this point, and Michelle seemed to convey a general unwillingness to have much to offer.

The therapist said that he would like to talk to them separately and asked who wanted to go first. The parents immediately asked to go first. Eric and Terry first wanted to get their anger and frustration off their chest about the day before. According to Eric and Terry, the HMO counselor interviewed them for 35 minutes before dismissing Michelle. During that 35 minutes, Eric and Terry shared their concerns regarding Michelle's suicidal expressions and her penchant for loudly defying Terry's requests for compliance to house rules. The HMO counselor listened without comment and began asking Michelle a series of questions about suicide. Michelle's answers were always yes with little or no elaboration. Michelle and the counselor never made eye contact, and Michelle did not share her views about anything.

After dismissing Michelle, the HMO counselor shared his conclusion that, based on his suicide lethality assessment, Michelle should be hospitalized immediately. The HMO counselor added that the situation was so serious that if the parents did not comply with his recommendation, then he would contact the county child protection agency.

Eric and Terry were both frightened for Michelle's safety and enraged by the HMO counselor's threat. They were pleased, however, that the new therapist was conducting separate interviews because they believed that Michelle did not feel comfortable talking in front of them—understatement, to say the least. The therapist proceeded to validate their experience of the day before in a variety of both verbal and nonverbal ways. The therapist was honestly amazed at the gross therapeutic blunder that had unfortunately been inflicted on this family. Here these concerned parents were looking for expert advice about a suicidal teenager (perhaps a parent's worst nightmare), and what they got was an ultimate invalidation in the form of a threat—not exactly an effective method for enlisting a cooperative working alliance.

The therapist was also astonished at the idea that an adolescent would not be interviewed separately as a matter of course. While this example offers a gross illustration in favor of separate interviews, which most therapists would likely do routinely, this kind of process on a more subtle level often occurs. That is, interviewing couples or families together only limits options and can sometimes squelch the open sharing required for validation and the coevolution of new meanings.

Eric and Terry seemed to be looking primarily for validation regarding their experience with the other counselor and for their daughter's lethality to be assessed by another professional. After thorough validation, the therapist brought Michelle in and sent the parents out.

The therapist asked Michelle what she was feeling suicidal about. She replied, "Everything." The therapist replied that things must have gotten real bad for her to consider killing herself as a solution, that people usually have to experience a lot of pain or be in a terrible situation to contemplate suicide.

Gradually, Michelle began talking, and her story unfolded. She was feeling suicidal and thinking of acting on it because she was under a lot of pressure at school and at home—at school because of gymnastics, and at home because her mother harassed her all the time about chores and rules. But on top of all that, she found out that her boyfriend had impregnated another girl. Michelle was devastated by his unfaithfulness, because he had told her that she was the only girl with whom he would ever have sex.

The therapist spent much of the rest of the interview validating Michelle's suicidal feelings, given all the pressures in her life and the recent discovery of her boyfriend's disloyalty. The therapist asked Michelle if she felt suicidal all the time, and she responded that she only felt suicidal when she was home and not when she was with her friends. The therapist pursued the exceptions and asked what about being home seemed to put her in a suicidal mode. Michelle responded that the main thing that made her suicidal was her mother. The therapist asked if that situation could be improved, then did Michelle think that her feelings of suicide would go away? Michelle replied, "Yes." The therapist responded by asking Michelle if: (1) she would be willing to put off killing herself to see if therapy could address that problem; and (2) she would be willing to call the therapist at any time if she felt like killing herself. Michelle answered in the affirmative. Finally the therapist asked if he could share their "contract" with Michelle's parents. Michelle agreed.

The therapist reunited the family and shared the no-suicide contract with the parents. The parents were validated and their fears assuaged by the no-suicide contract. Michelle's problem experience was similarly validated and seemed to enable her to agree to not only the contract, but also to address the problem with her mother. The interventions utilized in this case will be described in the next chapter. For now, consider how the separate interviews allowed: (1) Michelle to share her concerns uncensored (e.g., about her mother and her sexual involvement with her boyfriend); (2) validation of the parents and Michelle's experience without the risk of disconfirming anyone's point of view; and (3) the pursuit of Michelle's problem experience, which allowed for an exception to be noted (not suicidal when with friends) and a connection of the suicidal thoughts to her mother's harassment.

The Case of Sandra

To illustrate the main points of this chapter within one coherent example, the following edited transcript of a first interview will be presented with periodic commentary.

T: What brings you here to see me today?

C: I have had a few bad times of depression, real bad. I have had to fight real hard to keep things together, and a couple of times I got scared I would end up in the hospital. I wasn't handling things real well, so I thought, well rather than do that I'd better come and talk to you. You know, I don't feel that the medicine is helping me.

T: O.K. Sometimes it doesn't.

C: I felt like it had been up until the last month, you know, and then it just doesn't. I notice the big difference the way I had been handling things and I just, like I say maybe it's just me and maybe it is helping, but I don't feel it helping a lot.

T: How is your depression a problem for you?

C: Well, it just . . . I can go to bed and be fine and wake up the next morning, and it just is like the bottom has dropped out of everything and I just don't have any desire to live.

T: O.K.

C: I mean, it's just that bad that fast. I just . . .

T: So you can be O.K. the night before and when you wake up the next morning you just feel terrible.

C: Yes. *It is not like something happened and,* you know, *you get depressed over it,* you can't handle the problem. I just wake up that way and sometimes it lasts for days, several days, and I have to fight to keep going and *cry for no reason.* Everything is real hopeless.

T: During that time period—you say it lasts a few days?

C: Yes. Last weekend, I think, it lasted for 3 days and then . . . that's when I made the appointment. I was at work, but I had my daughter call to see if I could get an appointment to come over and talk to you, you know, because I got kind of scared because I thought I didn't want to be able to get help and not try to get it, so that's when I thought well, I felt, I was in trouble and better do something about it before it got the best of me.

T: Good. I am glad you felt that way and could prevent the hospitalization.

C: And I read all the papers, you know, that I got when I was in the hospital and when I have bad days I go over them but it just does not sink in.

T: It did not help. O.K.

C: You know it helped you then at the time, but it just doesn't . . . it just doesn't sink in to where you can grab it and get hold of yourself and go on.

T: What does it prevent you from doing that you want to do?

C: If I had . . . it's like you really have to fight to do everyday things like, you know, you go to work and you have to put up a front. It's like you put up a front like putting on your clothes in the morning and you really have to fight to keep that up because you don't want anybody to know that if I had my way about it, I would just kill myself and end it all. But really, you know, because I have the Lord and I know really He is the one that kept me going for a lot of years, so, you know, I have had to do a lot of praying and if it was not for my faith in Him, I would not have anything. But it just is real hard to do, to get up and go to work and put on this front and come home and you don't want to do anything, but you have to because you know you have a family. If I had my way, I would go to bed and stay there and never get up. I just want to go to sleep and not ever wake up, if I really had my way about it. That's just how I feel, you know, when I get that way. It's just kind of like a sadness inside that is always there. You just, you know, you look at other people—they can handle things, they seem happy and really, when you act like you are happy you are really putting up a front, because it is still there, you know, the sadness and the tension and I get tense and I cry all the time.

T: Now does this, when it comes, does it come every week for 2 or 3 days or is there a pattern to it?

C: No, there hasn't been. Sometimes, you know, I can go through 3 weeks and be able to handle things, I won't be depressed. I talk to myself,

"Don't let this problem get the best of you, handle it the best you can," and there isn't any pattern. That's why, I guess, I can understand it if something happened, if you had a problem and it caused you to get depressed. But, you know, I woke up yesterday morning, and it was just like the bottom had just fallen out of everything, and I was perfectly fine when I went to bed, at least I thought I was. I wasn't depressed or worried or anything and I just woke up that way and I can always . . . I thought, "Oh my, what am I getting up for?" and then you have to start fighting to be like you were yesterday.

T: How did you get up then? You mean you can make yourself do that?

C: Yes, I have learned to do that. You know, I have learned to kind of keep everything to myself as far as my job and everything goes. No one even knows why I was in the hospital. To the people I work with, they think I am the happiest person on earth, because I can do that just like putting on my shoes in the morning. You just kind of learn to do that, but on the inside you are not really happy and not really you. That's the way I see it.

T: So it is not really preventing you from doing anything, it is more of an internal kind of thing that you feel bad and sad about. O.K. And it happens just out of the blue and fairly regularly.

C: Yes, for the past months it has and it . . . I fought, you know, this for a long time as far as keeping me from doing anything and then even when I went and talked to the people at the Mental Health Center. I was still going to work and everything, but I knew I was in trouble. I knew I just couldn't handle things much longer, and that's kind of the way I am now. I mean, I don't want to go back to the hospital, so I told my husband last week I know I am in trouble, I can tell when it's getting the best of me. There was probably one whole spring when I did not do anything. I would just get up and sit there.

The therapist begins with questions designed to elicit an interactional description of the problem. In doing so, the client unfolds her meaning system regarding her depression. Her view is that the depression is an internally focused phenomenon unconnected to anything in her life circumstance. Notice the invalidation of her experience embedded in her expressions that are italicized.

T: So what have you tried so far to help yourself feel better, help yourself with your depression problem?

C: Well, I've certainly prayed a lot. That has helped, that always helps.

T: That always helps? So yesterday when you woke up—was it yesterday that you woke up?

C: Yesterday.

T: You prayed then?

C: Yes, all day. Lord, help me get through this day, help me do this, help me do that, just let me get through it. Like you could really care less about anything, you just don't care. You don't care about nothing and that is a terrible way to feel. You come home and you say, "*I should be happy. I have a nice home, my family loves me,*" and you think you could really care less, you don't care. How can you, you know, it's really hard to get up and do something or try to be interested in something. You think, I'll do this, it'll make me feel better, but it doesn't, and it's real hard to get yourself going when you just really don't care.

T: That kind of a general not caring is also part of your depression?

C: Yes.

T: You get kind of apathetic.

C: Yes.

T: O.K.—what else have you tried to help yourself? What kinds of things have you tried? What has your therapist suggested?

C: Doing something for yourself that would make you feel good. Spending time by yourself. Doing something for somebody else, but everything you think of you are not interested, you know, you just . . . and I have tried that, going to the store and getting something but you just really don't care, it does not make me feel any better.

T: So those things don't really help at all. Have you tried anything else?

C: No. I did get into the home interior business. I am doing that part-time. I really like that, I enjoy it. It's going to people's homes and having shows and selling pictures and things for the home, and I really enjoy that, and I felt really good about myself, you know, trying to kind of set a goal and reach it as far as that goes. But when I get depressed and everything, I just don't care. Even that does not help.

T: That doesn't help knowing that you have that to fall back on.

C: That is something that I really love to do, and I do it. It's helped give me self-confidence as far as being able to talk to people, because I am very . . . I don't like to talk to people at all, and it helps a lot just having the courage to go into somebody's home, and there are people there that you don't know and getting up and putting on a show. It has been real hard and I have done it, and I have felt good about it, but when I get depressed I know that doesn't even help me.

T: That doesn't help you either.

C: Nothing really makes me feel good about myself.

T: When you are feeling that way.

C: Yes, it's just such a hopeless feeling, you know. Everything you think of, it just doesn't matter. I really try to stay out of my family's way when I get that way, because it is real hard for them. It's real hard for them. It is as hard, probably, on them as it is on me.

T: How is it hard on them?

C: Because they really hate seeing me down and depressed, and I don't want to talk. Talking does not help, there just isn't anything that helps. You know, I go to bed early when I am like that, and they don't know what to do to make it better, and I don't know what to tell them, so I can see it's hard on them.

T: Yes.

C: Not understanding and not being able to help, so I usually stay out of everybody's way and you know it will pass and I will be O.K., and the next thing you know I am back where I started.

T: O.K.

C: It's just like a circle, and I think that I felt real good when I got out of the hospital. I did not feel that sadness inside, you know, and kind of down on myself, but then it just came back and it is probably my fault. I should have come a long time ago, *but I was real discouraged because my husband said he would come, but when it got down to it he didn't, and I got discouraged about that. I did not get depressed over it, I just got discouraged, you know.*

T: Well, you were hoping about him coming, and you two also working out some things.

C: That made a big difference, but he felt me coming, that would help me and there is not really anything that would help him, which I know is not true.

T: What has he suggested to you about ways of handling and getting over your depression problem?

C: Going out and doing something that I like to do, you know, he suggested to do what makes me happy. If I get up and don't feel like cleaning the house, don't worry about it, or do what I want to do—what makes me happy, but he doesn't understand that when you feel like that inside nothing makes you happy.

T: Mmm.

C: You know, I really don't think if someone gave me a million dollars when I feel that way it would make any difference. That is just . . . and that is a terrible attitude.

T: Well, it seems there is nothing anyone can do to make you happy at that point and time. You can't make yourself happy either.

C: There isn't. No, I certainly tried. You know, nobody wants to be like this.

T: No, nobody wants to be like that.

C: You are kind of tormented and tortured when you have all that turmoil going on inside, and you don't know what to do about it. The only thing I want to do when it's that bad is to go to sleep and not wake up. That's how I feel.

T: Have you been thinking about killing yourself?

C: No . . . Well, I probably would if it wasn't for the Lord. I really—I probably would do that.

T: O.K. But because of your faith, you won't do it?

C: No, because I am afraid of going to hell.

T: It does kind of eliminate your chances of getting into heaven.

C: Yes, that's why I said, "Lord, why can't I just lay down and go to sleep and you just take me on home, I don't see any purpose here." I know that's selfish.

T: But evidently he does have a purpose.

C: And you know, I know that's real selfish probably, and I wouldn't want to leave my kids and my husband, but it's just an example.

T: It's very hard not to think that way when you are in the pit. It is very difficult not to be selfish, because you are the one that is experiencing all the pain—nobody else is, and you just want the pain to stop, and that leads you to think those kinds of things.

C: That's what it is, you know, real torment and painful, and sometimes when it lasts for days, it's just all you can do, like I said, I have to do a lot of talking to myself, a lot of praying and really have a lot of faith. After it's over you are real exhausted mentally and physically. I just feel drained, just like I have been—I don't know what—for days without any sleep or any rest.

T: It takes a lot of psychic energy to be depressed.

C: Yes, it does.

T: It really drains you.

C: It does, that's the truth.

T: Mmm. Has he suggested other things to you as far as doing things that will help you feel better or help you not to be as depressed?

C: No.

T: No—has anybody else—friends or family or minister or . . . ?

C: No, I usually don't talk to anybody about it. I have one friend at work, you know, we go to church together and stuff, and I talk to her and she helped me a lot. I'm grateful for her being there to have someone to talk to, other than your husband, but no, I don't talk to anybody about it.

T: Yes.

C: I just want to be happy inside with me, and I know I can't change things around me all the time, you can't do things a lot of times about the problems, but you should be able to be happy yourself, *or to make things better as far as my husband and I. Maybe it bothers me and I don't realize it, but it just really isn't a real great factor any more.*

T: No?

C: No, it isn't. Because I know he has a problem, you know, that he can't help and until, I guess, he is ready to get help or whatever, then me being upset will not help things.

T: Now what's his problem?

C: He is impotent.

The therapist persistently pursued Sandra's solution attempts and those of others trying to help her. Many of the solutions were, of course, worthwhile, but were no longer helping. The interactional description of the problem was emerging as Sandra's feelings of depression, embedded in a cycle of Sandra trying to do things to make herself happy and others attempting to also get her to do things for herself. Doing things seemed to lead to Sandra experiencing that nothing was helping, that no matter what she did, she didn't have any impact on her depression (hopelessness), which led to more depression, which led to more attempts to influence her to take care of herself by doing things. "If nothing helps, and I have no reason to be depressed, I must really be bad off" seemed to be the client's view.

The questions also constructed an opportunity for meaning revision. As the story unfolded, the therapist continued asking questions within the content limitations presented by the client, until she brought up her husband's problem of impotence. The client had alluded to her husband earlier, and the therapist filed that information for future reference. When the client mentioned his problem, the door swung open, and the therapist walked through and pursued the path uncovered by the husband's impotence.

Many of the therapist's comments were validating ones. Note how a subtle shift occurred in the client's invalidation. Before, her comments were in the direction of there being no reason for her depression and that her husband's problem did not depress her. She begins to consider the possibility of the connection between her depression and his impotence in her comment, "Maybe it bothers me, and I don't realize it," but then quickly moves in the other direction.

T: You know, I am not trying to make you any more depressed by this, but a lot of people in relationships would certainly be depressed in relation to not having sex with their partner. I mean, sex is more than the sexual part of it, it is also a time when a man and a woman are intimate together emotionally. That's there to reaffirm their relationship, and it's there for those reasons as well; it's not just the sexual pleasure of it.

C: Right.

T: It's an intimate pleasure of it that keeps a marriage strong in a lot of ways. A lot of people certainly would be depressed or sad over not having that part of their life fulfilled.

C: Yes, it has been real hard, so I am not going to say it's been easy, and I wish things were different. I certainly do, *but as far as me thinking about it all the time or getting depressed over that, I don't.*

T: O.K. You know it is something that is there, but you don't spend a lot of time spinning your wheels over it.

C: Yes, because I have tried everything that I could think of, and it's not that he hasn't tried. It's just, I think, the fear of failure again that is just kind of a block there. I know he certainly has a problem, but for me to say, "You have a problem—do something about it," I am not going to tell anybody that.

T: No? Even though it's true?

C: Right. 'Cause you know, we have talked about it, and he doesn't feel it would do any good to come here.

T: I see, I see. O.K.

C: He doesn't feel like—what was it he said? Wait a minute—how did he say that? Something like, "when the time is right, it will happen—until then, there is just nothing you can do about it." I think that's a big cop-out.

T: Yes, I think it is too.

C: It is. I know it is something that he really can't help, just like he knows when I get depressed, it's something I really can't help. He has learned, you know, it's not really something that I can pull myself out of, pop myself out of, or whatever. So we really have a good understanding about each other's problems, I guess.

T: Sounds like it. I am amazed that you two have a good relationship based upon his problem and your problem, because it could ruin a lot of relationships.

C: Yes, it could. We were separated for a year, and he had an affair with another woman, and you know, I feel my depression had a lot to do with it, and so I did real good that year. I had all the kids, had all the responsibility, the house, I had it all just kind of dumped in my lap. I thought I did real good.

T: These things can really play havoc on a marriage, you know, and impotence can too, not that people are not understanding of it, but when it goes on and on it can be difficult.

C: It is hard. You know, there are a lot of times, some days, when I cannot even watch television. Where they have the soap operas and somebody is kissing or whatever, I just can't even watch. It bothers me, you know.

T: It makes you think about what you are not able to do.

C: Yes, it does. I am real careful about what I watch, you know, because I try to be careful not to let it get the best of me and, you know, you see something like that and you think, "Gosh, I wish we could be that way," and then you get to thinking about it and *I just try not to because it would probably cause me to get depressed or upset,* so I have to be real careful because it is hard, you know. Especially when you have had a good relationship and you know you love one another.

T: In other words, you get along pretty well.

C: Yes, we get along fine—we never fight or anything. At least if we fought, we could make up, but he won't fight.

T: You sometimes try to engage him in a fight, and he won't do it?

C: Yes, sometimes.

T: That's pretty frustrating too.

C: I know it.

T: Nothing worse than a person who won't fight with you.

C: I think, "Well, gosh, if he could get a little mad and fight, we could make up," but no, he doesn't like to fight. I don't know if that is a good marriage or not. They say people that never fight . . .

T: Well, you know fighting is part of being married.

C: Right.

T: And it usually means there is some closeness there, because you wouldn't fight unless you felt close because things wouldn't bother you. You would be apathetic about it. You would be like a roommate.

C: Yes, that's what it is like—a roommate.

T: No sex and no fighting. I don't know where you are getting that intensity from.

C: I don't know either, I really don't.

T: Because fighting and sex are a lot alike in that regard, because emotions are real intense then, and you are not having it either way.

C: No, we don't fight and we don't have sex, but there is something there that you know that each of you would never do anything to hurt the other and that you know that you both love one another, and you'd do anything to make that person happy that you could do. So, I don't know where it comes from, that's just about the way it is.

T: Is there ever any intensity between you two?

C: No, it is kind of like living with your roommate.

T: You've both got your jobs, your contribution to the household, and that kind of thing.

C: Yes, yes.

T: But not much like husband and wife.

C: No.

T: Because husband and wife—they *do* fight.

C: That's normal, you know, to get mad and fight. But, no, we don't fight. I think we have had one fight in the last year; it wasn't really a fight. We just, you know, had some words between us and, of course, the first thing he said was, "Well, you want me to leave?"

T: He pulled out the trump card, right?

C: Maybe he feels guilty, you know, when we were separated or whatever but I said, "No, I don't want you to leave," and then . . . I don't even know what we were fighting over now, but then he goes back in the living room and sits down, and I am in the kitchen, and we are both mad, and then he comes in and apologizes.

T: And it is over.

C: It is over, that's it. I think that's the only time in the past year that we have ever had words. No fighting and no sex—*no wonder I am depressed* [laughing].

T: Really. That's what I was thinking—no wonder you are depressed.

C: Well, it's better to laugh than cry.

T: Yes, yes. Although I think there is more to that than is funny. I think it may be an important factor of your depression.

C: I am sure it is. The way I look at it, that's the way the Lord made man and woman, you know, husband and wife.

T: Mmm.

C: And if He didn't want you to do those things, then you wouldn't have the desire for things that you have. So, therefore, knowing that, I came to the conclusion, you know, it's just not all there, you are not fulfilled, you are not all together. Because if it was not important, the way I feel about it, He wouldn't have made it so important in the Bible.

T: Mmm.

C: . . . from what I read and understand. So it is important.

T: Very important.

The opportunity emerged to unfold the client's story around her depression and cogenerate new or revised meanings around her depression. The conversation shifted from a description of an internally located and hopeless depression to a depression related to her longings for sexual intimacy with her husband, from a frame of reference offering little remedial action, other than what she was already trying unsuccessfully to help herself, to a frame of reference that perhaps could lead to a whole new set of options. The previously unspoken connection between her depression and her relationship was experienced by the client.

Notice how the conversation evolved to the point where the client replaced her own invalidation with the strong self-validation, "No wonder I am depressed." Validation of her own experience changed the tempo of the session, and Sandra's affect changed significantly from passive resignation to proactive involvement.

Sandra, as we will see in Chapter 6, confronted her husband and delivered an ultimatum, for the first time, that she would leave if he didn't seek help for his impotence. The case of Sandra illustrates the three aspects of the first interview. The therapist began by pursuing an interactional description of the client's depression. By doing so, the client's content-rich description unfolded her meaning system and presented an opportunity for meaning revision. The pursuit of an interactional description and the quest for revision opportunities allowed a context for the validation of the client's experience. Keeping the three levels in mind presents the therapist with a variety of change possibilities. If only validation occurs, the therapist is on the right track and may represent all that is needed by the client. If validation occurs, and an interactional description evolves, then an intervention can be co-constructed that extends the validation into the client's social environment. If validation occurs and a meaning revision opportunity emerges, then another possibility for change is available. Therapeutic openness and sensitivity to the rich field of unspoken and undiscovered avenues for rapid client change is perhaps the ideal characterization of a good therapist, which, hopefully, will continue to become manifest as we turn to the next chapters on intervention.

5   Suggesting Competing Experiences

THE common thread that unites the wide range of interventions that constitute competing experiences is the therapist's formulation of a direct suggestion that competes in some way with the client's actual experience of the presenting problem. The client's experience of the problem contains behavioral, cognitive, and affective components, thereby enabling the therapist to direct the suggestion at the component that the client emphasizes as significant. A competing experience, then, is *a suggestion that encourages an in vivo behavioral, cognitive, or affective competition with the client's current experience of the concern that served as the impetus for therapy.*

Competing experiences can take a myriad of forms ranging from general or abstract to specific or concrete, and can include tasks, rituals, prescriptions, direct suggestions, and homework assignments. Competing experiences include any technique from any theoretical orientation that the therapist asks the client to do, for example, relaxation exercises, journaling, natural consequences for child misbehavior, sensate focus, etc. In the context of the client's actual experience of the presenting problem, the client is asked to do, think, or feel something different than his or her usual experience of the problem.

In any given problem situation presented by a client, there are many possible competing experiences that could result in problem improvement. A plethora of techniques are readily available to the interested therapist. Strategically oriented authors such as Haley, Madanes, the MRI, Selvini-Palazzoli, de Shazer, Weiner-Davis, and O'Hanlon have contributed to a literature that is rich in alternative experiences that may be utilized. (See Appendix A for a list of possible competing experiences.) The problem, of course, is not a dearth of possible interventions or a paucity of plausible competing experiences, but the lack of a coherent system through which competing experiences can be designed to meet the unique client situation under concern.

This chapter presents the clinical application of suggesting competing experiences, and provides guidelines for selection, design, delivery, and follow-through. A method of selection flowing from three considerations and specific criteria for the design of competing experiences based in the multilevel description of the change process (Pragmatic Assumption #3) will be introduced. The three general considerations emphasize the importance of a resource-based perspective and speak to the process the therapist employs to select options for intervention. The multilevel description of change serves as a framework for suggesting competing experiences specifically tailored to the particulars of the client's idiosyncratic presentation.

SELECTING COMPETING EXPERIENCES: GENERAL CONSIDERATIONS

People who enter therapy, except in certain compulsory situations, do so because the experience of their lives or some specific circumstance has become so painful or distressing that a change of some kind is perceived as necessary. Clients may initially appear frustrated and helpless, creative energies may be at a low ebb, and the perception may exist that they have tried everything possible only to have experienced failure time after time. The client's frustration and helplessness should be respected by the therapist and not considered as a reflection of any deficits or psychopathology.

Dependence on the Client's Resources

The initial consideration for the therapist is to maintain a nonpathology frame as suggested in Pragmatic Assumption #1 (i.e., the problem, and its solution, are embedded in the interactive process.) Such a frame is critical to the design of competing experiences because the therapist is counting on the existent resources and strengths of the client. Competing experiences offer opportunities for change that promote clients utilization of their own inherent capacities for growth. A pathology frame may undermine the therapist's confidence in the resources of clients and, therefore, limit the range of competing experiences from which to choose. An initial consideration, then, is the recognition that competing experiences depend upon the resources of clients.

Lynn

Recall Lynn, who was convinced that her daughter's irritability and unhappiness were signs of a genetically transmitted depression. (See Appendix B for page numbers.) Lynn was taking both antipsychotic and antidepressant medications and had been under psychiatric care for 9 years. Pathology frames were readily available in Lynn's presentation. The therapist, however, did not adopt a pathology frame, but instead pursued the selection of a competing experience that depended on Lynn's resources. Lynn found within herself the strength to alter her parenting style with her daughter.

As an aside, it is interesting to note that Lynn recontacted the therapist shortly after termination. Lynn wanted to know whether the therapist thought that she needed to be on antipsychotics. The therapist replied that Lynn did not seem psychotic to him. The therapist consulted with the psychiatrist, and Lynn ultimately discontinued antipsychotic medication. Depending on the resources of clients sets the stage for clients to utilize their inherent capacity for growth.

What the Client Wants

The next general consideration in selecting competing experiences is that the intervention must address what the client defines as problematic and what the client indicates as the goals for therapy, as suggested in Pragmatic Assumption #2 (i.e., the client's presentation, rather than the therapist's orientation, determines therapy goals, the content of the therapeutic conversation, and intervention strategies.) Rather than an imposition of the therapist's theoretical (or personal) frame of reference, the competing experience is a response to the client's formulation of the problem experience. The client's desires, therefore, set the focus and structure of the selection process.

Selecting competing experiences begins by accepting the client's presentation at face value, without any reformulation, and then matching that general presentation of the problem situation (e.g., parent–child conflict, marital problem, depression, anxiety, etc.) with rationales and treatment options for the particular problem area that are available to the therapist. Such rationales and treatment options may emerge from the therapist's previous experiences, the literature, workshops, or some creative combination. This aspect of selection is limited only by the therapist's resources and knowledge base. The second consideration, then, is characterized by an explicit therapist acceptance of what the client wants and a start of a general search for intervention options that directly address the client's desires.

Lynn

Lynn's presentation of the problem (her daughter's genetic depression) and what she wanted from therapy (suggestions regarding how to help her daughter) was accepted at face value and served as the basis for a beginning search for possible interventions. Lynn's general presentation generated the following options for the selection of a competing experience: suggestions flowing from a low self-esteem perspective of Amy's depression (e.g., building self-esteem); suggestions based in a view of the depression as related to Lynn's relationship with her husband (e.g., marital therapy; pretend assignments, Madanes, 1981; odd/even rituals, Selvini-Palazzoli, Boscolo, Cecchin, & Prata, 1978); suggestions based in a behavior modification frame of reference (e.g., differential reinforcement of competing behaviors, Redd, Porterfield, & Anderson, 1979); and suggestions based in an interactional/solution focused perspective (e.g., encouraging expression of depression, Watzlawick et al., 1974); "inviting what you dread" (Duncan & Rock, 1991); formula tasks (de Shazer, 1985). Other possible considerations were individual/play therapy for Amy and pharmacotherapy. Accepting the client at face value and initiating an intervention search based upon client desires leads to the final general aspect of selection, namely, the collaborative exploration of options that fit the client's idiosyncratic experience of the problem.

Collaborative Exploration

The final consideration is that selection is a collaborative exploration process that emerges from the therapist–client conversation and the clients' articulation of their content-rich meaning system. From clients' general presentations, the therapist has several intervention options in mind. As clients tell their problem stories, they elaborate the idiosyncrasies of their experiences, their views of the problem itself and perhaps how it may be best approached, and what they have tried previously to do to solve the problem. These elaborations by clients enable a co-selection of interventions that seem congruent with clients' experiences of their problems. The therapist contributes to the narrowing of options by introducing different rationales for treatment approaches through the dialogue about the problem. The therapist essentially sends up trial balloons to explore the clients' responses regarding the relevancy of a given intervention option.

The client, then, collaborates in the selection process during the interview in two ways. First, just by virtue of the client's description of the problem experience, the therapist continuously evaluates the multiple options and begins to rule out choices that are obviously antithetical to the client's meaning system. Second, clients respond to treatment rationales introduced by the therapist, and, on the basis of client's receptivity to the rationales, the therapist proceeds with those options or discards them.

The client can also collaborate in the design of the intervention outside of therapy. If the therapist is uncertain about which intervention or set of interventions to pursue, then the therapist can enlist the client's help by asking the client to do one of several variations on the theme of observing the problem experience or observing the experience of not having the problem (de Shazer, 1985; O'Hanlon & Weiner-Davis, 1989). Such generic or formula interventions are often helpful when the therapist has been unable to gain enough information to eliminate treatment options and does not want to suggest a specific competing experience without further exploration of the client's meaning system surrounding the problem. Observe tasks are also useful as parsimonious and unintrusive attempts to enable the possibility for change. The client's experience of the observe task serves to enable a further evaluation and co-selection process. The formula tasks also promote revision experiences that may render other interventions unnecessary.

Lynn

As the therapeutic conversation unfolded, Lynn and the therapist began the process of collaborative exploration of treatment options. Lynn reported that she was a "stroker" and spent much time and effort rewarding Amy and attempting to build her low self-esteem. This included inventing games to play, praising Amy at every opportunity, and completing a self-esteem workbook that Lynn obtained from a school counselor. Based upon this report, the therapist no longer considered options based on self-esteem or behavior modification. Lynn also indicated that she would prefer to address Amy's depression without medication, if possible, and that was why she did not approach her own psychiatrist for help.

The therapist suggested that some therapists believe that child problems are sometimes related to marital conflict and asked Lynn if that made any sense to her. Lynn responded that yes, it made sense to her, but not in her case because she had a wonderful marriage and a wonderful husband. Consequently, the topic of the client's marriage was dropped as quickly as it was introduced. Intervention options based on that rationale were also dropped.

Based upon the narrowing of options just described and on the strongly held client meaning of "genetic depression," the therapist selected the "diathesis-stress" model as a content area and suggested a competing experience based upon an interactional/solution-focused perspective. The therapist discussed the importance of the environmental aspect of genetic predispositions and suggested that Lynn encourage her daughter's negative expressions, validate them, and perhaps even exaggerate them as a way to help her work through her feelings and learn to cope with her depressive tendencies. Lynn responded very positively to the suggestion and expressed her willingness to try the different approach. The competing experience evolved from a collaborative exploration and elimination of treatment options through the client's articulation of her experience and the therapist's introduction of different rationales.

Lynn reported that Amy was much better and was smiling more (the negotiated sign of improvement). Lynn added that she realized how she was rescuing her daughter from her depression and that Amy would be better off to work through things, with Lynn's support, on her own. Lynn was pleased to conclude that perhaps Amy was only *mildly* predisposed to depression. Finally, Lynn also indicated that she had fun with the exaggerate part of the suggestion. On several occasions, Lynn had exaggerated Amy's negative comments to such an extreme degree that both of them broke out laughing.

DESIGNING COMPETING EXPERIENCES: THE MULTILEVEL DESCRIPTION OF CHANGE

From the level of change that pursues an interruption of the problem cycle, competing experiences are designed to interdict current unsuccessful solution attempts. Viewing change from a perspective of meaning revision, competing experiences are designed to provide a contextual competition with the client's experience of the problem to enable the opportunity for the creation of new meanings. Finally from a common factors description of change, competing experiences are designed to explicitly validate the client's meaning system and extend the interpersonal context of the relationship to the client's social environment. Competing experiences therefore involve a dynamic interplay of technique and relationship that are experiential enactments of the therapeutic alliance outside of therapy. Competing experiences extend the quest for change opportunities to the time between sessions. Within each level of change there are criteria that contribute to the specific design of competing experiences.

Interrupting Solution Attempts

According to the MRI (Fisch et al., 1982) problems occur within a context of behavior. In a broad sense, behavior may be described as actions related to thinking, feeling, or doing. Within this behavioral context, each person's behavior instigates and structures the behavior of others and vice versa. When people are in contact over time, repetitive patterns or cycles of interaction develop. In the situation in which a problem arises, attempts to resolve the problem become a part of an interactional cycle. Attempted solutions form a relationship with the problem so that the more the problem behavior is exhibited, the more attempted solutions are applied. Attempted solutions that fail to produce a desired change become the impetus for more problem behavior. Simultaneously, increasing problem behavior becomes the impetus for more solution attempts. Recall Mark from Chapter 4. Mark's problem of concentration and worry occurred in a problem cycle consisting of a variety of efforts to reassure and browbeat himself, which decreased his ability to concentrate, which led to more worrying and more reassurance from others, and so on.

The MRI also suggests that any interruption of the solution pattern, be it stopping the client's current solution attempts or initiating a solution that is appreciably different from the solutions being employed, will result in a change or shift in the problem cycle. The competing experience, then, may be designed from the consideration of two questions: (1) What can the client do that will stop the current solution attempts? (2) What other solutions can be suggested that run counter to the solutions currently employed? The competing experience designed for Mark consisted of asking him to observe the differences between when he was able to concentrate at school with his classmates and when he was at home and didn't concentrate as well, and to pay particular attention to how he was able to overcome his worry and focus his concentration (see de Shazer, 1985). In designing the competing experience, the therapist considered what would stop Mark's solutions of reassurance and self-criticism and what Mark could do that would run counter to his current unsuccessful solution attempts. The competing experience was ultimately designed to stop Mark's worrying, browbeating, and surface reassurances by shifting the focus toward how he was already successfully concentrating.

Mary

Mary, a 37-year-old housewife, sought therapy because of a marital problem. Her husband had recently begun coming home late and going out for long periods of time at night. Several telephone calls in which the other party hung up after Mary answered resulted in Mary's considering the possibility that her husband was having an affair. Mary began restricting trips out of the home because she wanted to "be there" for her husband. She brought up the possibility of an affair with her husband, but he both denied an affair and accused Mary of attempting to control his comings and goings. A cycle of interaction evolved in which Mary held a vigil at home waiting anxiously for her husband. With increasing frequency, Mary brought up the accusation that her husband was having an affair, and, in response, her husband became more vehement about his right to go where he pleased.

Thinking about the pattern of Mary's solution attempts and her husband's response, the therapist considers: (1) What can Mary do to stop waiting on her husband and cease accusations, and (2) what can she do that would run counter to these attempts to solve the marriage problem? With these questions in mind, the therapist suggests that Mary make herself less available to her husband. Unavailability would include making some trips out of the house, particularly when her husband is home, or about to arrive, and waiting for her husband to initiate discussion about where he has been or why he is late. This experience is suggested to Mary because making herself less available and going out of the house runs counter to waiting for him and staying near the house. Avoiding the initiation of discussion about where he has been also stops the problem cycle of Mary accusing and her husband denying (Fisch et al., 1982).

From the level of change that views strategy as interrupting the behavioral interaction that constitutes the problem cycle, the competing experience is designed to stop the current solution patterns and/or shift the client in a significantly different direction from the basic thrust of the unsuccessful attempted solutions. This level attempts to influence the client to simply do something (or stop doing something) regarding the problem so that the problem cycle is jammed, and a new cycle of behavioral interaction can emerge.

Meaning Revision

Based in the level of change that seeks to interrupt the problem cycle, competing experiences serve to either block the client's current solution strategies or initiate alternative solutions. Such a therapeutic thrust is a useful place to start, but additional factors revolving around meaning formation and maintenance provide further guidance in the design of competing experiences. Considering the meaning system surrounding the client's experience of the problem enables a tailored design of an intervention, such that the therapist's suggestion becomes a uniquely constructed competing *meaning* experience.

People continually evolve meaning systems through dynamic social exchange and their capacity to rehearse and process social interaction before and after its occurrence. Once a situation acquires a meaning of "problem," a complex set of interactions between meaning and behavior emerges. The meanings ascribed to problematic circumstances carry implicit structures or rules that have a direct impact on solutions that are perceived as reasonable to apply. The ascribed meanings carry a compelling logic based upon the success of similar meanings in past interactions, as well as other experiences with the family, subculture, or larger cultural setting. Regardless of their developmental and contextual history, the meanings attributed to the problem influence what remedial actions are chosen, and those actions either confirm or revise those meanings in a reciprocal fashion.

Meanings that evolve from interaction around a problem sometimes become reified, forming a cycle with experience that inadvertently empowers meanings that bring pain and distress. These problem meaning systems may be deconstructed and revised when a therapist makes a suggestion that encourages an in vivo behavioral, cognitive, or affective competition with the client's current experience of the problem. Such a contextual competition enables the client to challenge the limitations of the problem meaning system and permits the opportunity for the creation of new meanings.

Although a certain degree of spontaneity and creativity is helpful when designing competing experiences, the therapist's determination of the client's emphasis on either affective, cognitive, or behavioral aspects of the problem provides a pragmatic criterion for further specificity of the intervention. As the therapeutic conversation unfolds, clients describe their informal theories and, in doing so, provide guidance regarding the most salient components of the problem experience, that is, clients generally emphasize their experiences of the problem as being primarily behavioral, cognitive, or affective. Using the client's emphasis as a guide (not as a hard and fast rule), the therapist may then design a competing meaning experience that contains a new component that not only changes the context of how the problem is experienced, but also specifically competes with the most salient aspect of that experience as described by the client. Such a focused contextual competition promotes opportunities for revision of meaning and, therefore, prompts an emergent meaning system that is less distressing and permits alternative solution strategies.

Assessing the Primary Emphasis

To develop a focus that zeros in on the primary emphasis of the client's problem experience, the therapist may consider the following questions: (1) How does the client present the concern itself? (2) Is it a problem of behavior or something that the client (or someone else) is doing that is distressing? (3) Is it a problem of cognition, or something that the client is thinking that is of concern? (4) Is it a problem of affect, or something that the client is feeling that is troubling? (5) How does the client describe what change will look like? (6) Will change be experienced by feeling, thinking, or behaving differently?

Frequently, clients will provide this information without being directly asked. The therapist then needs only to remember and organize this information. "Johnnie is so belligerent. All we ever do is yell at one another." "George needs to do something to show that he really cares." "I can't stop myself from thinking about my mother's death." Statements like these not only create a sense of what is meaningful to the client, but also help shape the therapist's thinking when designing a task or homework assignment. The pragmatic assumption that the client's presentation, rather than the therapist's orientation, determines the intervention is enacted when the competing meaning experience matches the expressed emphasis of the client.

Looking for the most salient aspect of the problem experience from the client's point of view is distinguished from approaches that place an invariant value on one component of the experience over another. For example, placing an invariant value on affect or cognition when such a value is contradictory to the client's presentation runs the risk of undermining the alliance and, therefore, positive outcome. Just as standby reflections of feeling do not address the empathic needs of many clients, placing an invariant value on feelings, thoughts, or behaviors will similarly miss the boat with many clients.

The common therapist belief that people who express their feelings are healthier than those who express their experiences in cognitive terms is another example of not only a subtle deficit view of clients (i.e., people who do not express feelings are not in touch), but also a therapist or orientation value that is imposed on clients that often does not fit. The perspective addressed here, on attending to the client's emphasis, is intended merely as a guide for shaping competing meaning experiences; one emphasis is not viewed as any better than another.

Mark and Mary

Recall Mark and the therapist's suggestion that Mark observe the differences between when he was able to concentrate and when he was not, paying attention to how he was able to overcome his worrying. In addition to interrupting Mark's solution attempts, the intervention was designed based on Mark's description of the problem as primarily cognitive, that is, involving concentration and worrying. The competing meaning experience was primarily cognitive and therefore competed directly with the problem experience most emphasized by the client. Placing the client and the problem in a new context creates the opportunity for meaning revision. Mark returned and stated that his concentration and worry problems were greatly exacerbated by a lack of sleep and that he now thought that if he could get a good night's sleep, things would be a lot better. Mark's connection of his problem to a lack of sleep occurred in a context of competition between old and new ways of cognitively experiencing his problem. This enabled Mark to challenge the limitations of his meaning system and arrive at a conclusion that permitted a different set of solution options. The revision occurred via Mark's cognitively altered experience. We will return to the therapist's response in the follow-through section.

Recall Mary and the suggested competing experience offered by the therapist. Another dimension of the design of the intervention arose from Mary's behavioral description of the problem and her stated goals. In addition to Mary's behavioral presentation of her attempts to solve the problem, she also disclosed that her main hope was for her husband to return to his "normal behavior." Her accusations of an affair and staying close to home were not based on finding out what her husband was really doing, but rather predicated on the hope that she would attract her husband's attention and get him to come home as he once did. Mary also stated that staying home and accusing her husband constituted her way of doing something to save the marriage. She just could not bear to "sit back and not do anything."

The suggestion to make herself less available (go out more, particularly when her husband was expected to be home) was not only suggested to interrupt Mary's attempts at solving the problem, but also to do so in a manner that was consistent with her behavioral description of the problem and her goals. Such a contextual competition sets the stage for revisions of meaning to occur. Mary enacted the suggestions, and her husband began staying out less and attending more to Mary's needs. Her husband began wondering about what Mary was doing. The "affair" was no longer discussed. Mary ultimately concluded that perhaps she had become a little too reliant on her husband and continued to engage in more outside social activity. The revision of meaning occurred in a context in which a competition between old and new ways of addressing her problem enabled both Mary and her husband to reevaluate the limitations of their meaning systems.

Janice

Mark is illustrative of a client who presented with a cognitive focus, and Mary as one who described her situation in primarily behavioral terms. Consider Janice, who presented an affective emphasis concerning her fear of flying. Janice was a 32-year-old executive recently promoted to a position that required her to fly to regional meetings. She reported that she had successfully avoided flying for many years to the point of leaving situations in which flying was discussed or even overheard on television. Janice described her fears as extreme feelings of panic and a most distressful feeling of going crazy. She wanted to feel in control of her fears and to diminish her fear to a degree that she could fly to her regional meetings. Janice added that she believed her fears were an overreaction, given how most people fly without feeling much fear.

Janice presented her concern in both affective and cognitive terms, although her primary emphasis was on *feeling* in control and *feeling* less fear. Based upon Janice's affective emphasis, the therapist employed a symptom prescription and suggested that Janice spend at least 15 minutes, but not more than 30 minutes, considering the dangers of flying and feeling her fears intensely. To this point of our discussion, the symptom prescription or competing experience was designed to: (1) interrupt the client's current solution attempts revolving around the theme of avoidance; and (2) create an experience or construct a context that competed affectively with her feelings of being out of control by placing her in control, thereby creating an opportunity for an in vivo challenge of her meaning system that her fears were an overreaction and were uncontrollable.

Janice returned and reported that her fears seemed more manageable, which was followed by a lengthy discussion of all the dangers that Janice thought of during the prescription. Janice added that she talked to other people about her flying fears (for the first time) and discovered that others, to her surprise, felt afraid also. The therapist concluded the discussion with another competing experience that was in the form of a specific task. After asking Janice if she was willing to participate in an experiment and getting her agreement, the therapist asked Janice to go to the airport and observe ten people awaiting departure and rate their anxiety levels on a scale of 1 to 10. We will return to Janice's experience of this suggestion in the next section. Janice's sense of being able to better manage her fear emerged from a competition between old and new ways of affectively experiencing her flying fears. The revision of meaning evolved from Janice's affectively altered experience, which led to different solution alternatives such as talking to others about their fears of flying.

Competing meaning experiences are not directed toward the client arriving at a particular revision in meaning that the therapist has specifically in mind. Rather, competing experiences merely provide the opportunity for revisions to occur and, therefore, rely on inherent resources of the client and the human tendency to attribute meaning to experience. The therapist did not expect Mark to discover that his concentration was directly related to a sleep problem, Mary to conclude that she was too reliant on her husband and needed to act independently on her own behalf, or Janice to experience her fears as more manageable and seek others' opinions about flying. All three instances arose from competing experiences that placed a great deal of faith in the individual's capacity to grow and resolve problems.

Validation Through Competing Experiences

Competing experiences have been discussed as providing interruptions of the problem cycle and as methods of constructing opportunities through contextual competition to enable the generation of new or revised meanings. Competing experiences, however, are more than solution interruptions or meaning revision opportunities. Competing experiences provide a vehicle through which the interpersonal context of the relationship can be extended to the client's social environment.

Competing experiences can offer in vivo validation of the client's meaning system that supports the client in risking a revision of meaning or change in the problem circumstance. Competing experiences, therefore, represent a combination of technique and relationship that are experiential enactments of the therapeutic alliance. By working toward the goals defined by the client and focusing specifically upon the primary emphasis of the client's problem experience, competing experiences are also designed to include a validation of both the client's desire to change and the meaning system surrounding the presenting problem.

Validating the desire for change and the client's meaning system is the last criterion to consider when designing a competing experience. The suggestion of competing experiences without validation (as perceived by the client) generally results in unfortunate outcomes such as the client not enacting the suggestion or returning with the problem remaining the same or even worsened.

Validation and Saving Face

One way of further understanding the criterion of validation in addition to the common factors rationale is provided by the contributions of Milton Erickson (1980). Erickson believed that people are naturally protective of their failed solution efforts and the meanings associated with them. Consequently, persons entering therapy are considered to have both the desire to change and a natural inclination to protect themselves if movement toward change threatens personal dignity. In this way, problem meaning systems are maintained, not only by repeated failed solution attempts, but also by the threat that dignity will be lost if change necessitates admission of the incorrectness of one's premises and the corresponding meaning system.

Many have viewed this human inclination as a phenomenon to be analyzed and worked through. In contrast, Erickson argued that the need to preserve dignity can be effectively addressed by the therapist in the service of the client's desired change. Erickson might say that clients require the therapist to provide a face-saving space for the client to risk taking steps toward change. Said another way, clients who are explicitly validated by the therapeutic relationship are free to use their own resources unencumbered by the invalidation of their own or others' descriptions of their concerns.

Recall that validation reflects a combination of the therapist varia-bles of empathy, respect, and genuineness. The therapist genuinely accepts the client's presentation at face value, the therapist respects the client's experience of the problem by highlighting its importance, and the thera-pist empathically offers total justification of the client's experience. Validation is considered to be so essential to the success of therapy that it should be incorporated in all phases of therapy: in the session, in the delivery of the competing experience, and in the competing experience itself.

Validation can be difficult, and the therapist may sometimes need to challenge him- or herself to maintain an attitude that clients are doing the best they can under the circumstances. Sometimes it is helpful to think of the presenting problem as representing some form of intrinsic wisdom, or benefiting the client in some way, or any other meaning that will enhance therapist ability to validate the client's experience without attributions of deficits or pathology.

Creating Validating Experiences

Competing experiences provide validation of the client's desire for change quite simply by addressing the goals defined by the client and by targeting the most salient aspect of the client's problem experience. Providing validation of the meaning system associated with the presenting problem is a little more complicated and may be accomplished in two ways. One way is the presentation of the competing experience within a larger frame that validates the client's meaning system. The other way is designing the competing experience itself in such a way that it contains an inherent validation.

Likewise, presenting the competing experience within a larger frame that validates the client's meaning system may be achieved in a couple of ways. One way entails discussing the useful purposes of the client's problem, the advantages they may bring, or the disadvantages that may arise from problem resolution, thereby validating the client's reasons for not already changing and/or justifying the difficulty the client has encoun-tered in his or her attempts to resolve the problem. Such discussions validate the experience of ambivalence about change (the MRI would call this the "dangers of change" and promote its use for different reasons).

John had suffered with agoraphobia for several years and had been in therapy for about 3 years when his therapist moved out of town. The new therapist wanted to suggest a competing experience in the form of asking John to construct a desensitization hierarchy of things he would like to accomplish on a scale of least difficult to most difficult. The therapist engaged John in a discussion around the useful aspects of his agoraphobia and some possible drawbacks to changing it. John identified that his agoraphobia enabled him to pursue his favorite hobbies of antique refinishing and reading, and that if he were to improve or change the agoraphobia, he might have to accept a less than ideal job situation.

With each topic that arose in the conversation, the therapist provided validation of the client's predicament, given the benefits of the problem and the risks of attempting to change it. After a lengthy discussion, the therapist suggested the competing experience. John was then in a position to experience the assignment as a between-session extension of a context that validated his meaning system about the problem and his desire for change. John returned, having constructed the hierarchy, and to the utter astonishment of his therapist, accomplished the most difficult item on his list. The intervention arose from a context of validation of John's difficulty in changing his agoraphobia. The intervention promoted the alliance because the client goals were accepted at face value, and the task itself flowed directly from the client's experience.

The other way of presenting an intervention within a larger frame that contains validation entails simply highlighting the validation that has already occurred in the session by further emphasizing the significance of the client's problem, the importance of the struggle he or she is facing, and total justification of the client's idiosyncratic manifestation of the problem. Such a larger frame often is in a form similar to this statement: "Because of all these things that have happened to you and all the distress that you have suffered, I want to ask you to consider engaging in an experiment that may help us both to learn more about the problem and how it may be improved." The competing experience is presented in a way that sets a cause–effect connection between the validation and the intervention itself.

Before presenting the competing experience to Mark, the therapist reiterated the importance of Mark's concentration and worry, and the complete legitimacy of Mark's feelings of depression, given that school represented success or failure in life to Mark. Mark's own internal invalidation ("I shouldn't worry, this is stupid!") and others' discounting of his distress ("You'll do fine, you always have before") was replaced with a validation message that better matched his feelings of depression. The therapist's comments were more congruent with Mark's actual experience of his concentration problem. The therapist said:

"Because of what your returning to school means to you, that this is essentially a do or die test of how you are going to think of yourself the rest of your life, I want to ask you not to minimize the significance of this problem. Rather, to focus more on your concentration ability by observing the difference between when you are able to concentrate at school and when you are home and don't do as well. Pay particular attention to how you are able to overcome your worry and concentrate better."

The competing experience, which validated Mark's desire for change by addressing his goals for therapy, was directly linked to the validation of Mark's concern as significant and his feelings of depression as justified. The intervention then represented an explicit therapist behavior that not only demonstrated empathy, respect, and genuineness, but also extended the relational context of validation to the client's social environment.

Designing the competing experience itself in such a way that it contains an inherent validation is not as difficult as it may appear. A competing experience is the behavioral manifestation of the relationship and its effectiveness depends on the meaning given to it in the context of therapy. Competing experiences that are designed as suggestions based in the client's meaning system are inherently validating, because the intervention demonstrates the therapist's acceptance of the client's meaning each time the client enacts the suggestion. Each time a suggestion is attempted, the alliance is extended to the client's natural world. Validation, once experienced, may allow clients the support and freedom to risk a revision of meaning about their concerns. Out-of-session validation is very powerful and perhaps may be the most important aspect of encouraging clients to utilize their own strengths to resolve problems.

An example of an intervention that provided between-session validation of the client's meaning system can be found in the case of Mary. Mary's meaning system regarding her husband's recent behavioral changes revolved around a strongly held value to save the marriage. Validating Mary's resolve to save her marriage became an important component in the design of a competing experience. The therapist accepted Mary's presentation of her marital problem, respected the value she placed on saving her marriage, and suggested an intervention that flowed from that value.

Mary was quite relieved when the therapist ascribed no special meaning or fault to her desire to save the marriage. Prior to calling the therapist, she confided in a friend who told Mary that she was foolish for not making more of the affair. The friend advised Mary to seek evidence of the affair by having her husband followed, and then file for divorce.

The friend also implied that Mary was co-dependent to be so eager to remain in such a bad marriage.

The therapist did not question the wisdom in saving the marriage, but rather validated Mary's desire to keep the marriage together, given the length of the marriage and her previously experienced contentment with most aspects of the relationship. The therapist extended the in-session validation to Mary's natural environment by an intervention that validated Mary's meaning system every time she enacted the suggestion to make herself less available. Each time she left the house or waited for her husband to initiate conversation, Mary was doing so in service of saving the marriage. The competing experience interrupted her unsuccessful solution attempts, created an opportunity for meaning revision through Mary's behaviorally altered interaction with her husband, and validated her meaning system regarding saving the marriage.

Janice

Symptom prescription (asking the client to engage in the very problem attempting to be changed) can also be designed in certain client situations to contain a validation within the prescription itself. Recall Janice and her feelings of being out of control, and her statement that her fears constituted an overreaction to flying. Janice not only experienced the distress of her fears and a resultant inability to fly, but also the indignity of not being able to control her feelings. Janice seemed embarrassed about her fears as evidenced by her view that they were an overreaction and by her previous reluctance to discuss her fears with anyone else. Janice's description of her fears contained her own invalidation of her experience. Note the incongruence between Janice's experience of extreme distress and her view that her distress was an overreaction, that is, not valid or an exaggeration of something that was really trivial. The prescription, therefore, was designed not only to interrupt her avoidance and promote meaning revision, but also to validate Janice's distress as legitimate.

The therapist presented the prescription as part of a larger frame that validated Janice's experience by briefly discussing the inherent dangers and risks associated with hurling through space at 30,000 feet in a 20-ton metal cylinder going 600 miles an hour. Janice was asked to take the first step toward control through deliberately making her fears intense by thinking of the risks of flying. The intervention not only supported Janice's desire for more control, but also validated her fears as completely justified and legitimate, given the obvious dangers of flying. The competing experience extended the relational context of validation into the client's natural environment, which seemed to support Janice in revising her meaning system regarding her fears.

Janice returned having experienced more control and having discussed flying fears with others. The discussion of the dangers of flying further legitimatized Janice's fears, and the conversation evolved to a point in which the therapist suggested that many people have fears about flying and that he, too, experienced high anxiety during takeoff and landing. The therapist further validated the legitimacy of Janice's fears and highlighted the significance of Janice's newly found evidence that others were also uncomfortable by suggesting another competing experience.

The airport rating exercise was specifically designed to continue validating Janice's experience of her fears as justifiable. Janice returned and reported surprise that seven out of ten people observed had ratings of six or more, and she was pleased that not everyone took flying in stride as she once thought. The competing experience also represented a continued interruption of the solution attempt of avoidance as well as continued opportunity for meaning revision. Perhaps more important, once Janice no longer experienced invalidation of her distress, she was able to pursue improvement of her problem. Therapy also included a relaxation exercise to help Janice control her fears, and termination occurred after Janice's first successful, although very uncomfortable, flying experience.

Selecting and Designing
Competing Experiences: Summary

There are three selection considerations for choosing interventions. First is the recognition that competing experiences depend upon the client's resources. Pathology frames may undermine and limit the selection process. Next is the explicit therapist acceptance of what the client requests from therapy and a start of a general search for treatment options that directly address the client desires. The final consideration presents the overall process as a collaborative exploration of treatment options that evolves from the therapeutic dialogue and the clients' elaboration of the problem experience. The multilevel description of change provides three criteria as guidelines for designing competing experiences. First, the intervention should interrupt the client's current solution attempts by either blocking them or initiating a solution appreciably different. Second, the therapist suggestion should match the primary emphasis the client places on either the affective, behavioral, or cognitive experience of the problem. Such a suggestion enables a competing meaning experience in which an in vivo reevaluation and revision of meaning can occur. Finally, the competing experience should be designed to both validate the client's meaning system regarding the problem and the client's desire for change.

Recently, a number of authors (e.g., Hoffman, 1985, Goolishian & Anderson, 1992) have criticized and deemphasized homework assign- ments and have refocused the locus of change on the interview process. This shift in focus has been very helpful in our consideration of the many opportunities for change that arise in the interview through the mutual exploration of meaning and the validation of the client's experience. The shift of focus to the interview has put homework assignments and tasks in perspective. Overemphasis on developing "clever" interventions may result in the therapist's not attending to the client and missing opportunities for client-initiated changes during the interview.

On the other hand, well-constructed interventions that emerge from and punctuate significant aspects of the interview process can extend the quest for change opportunities and the validation context of the relationship to between sessions as well. We believe that dismissing the possibilities for between-session opportunities for change because of a view that homework assignments are "too instrumental" is a limiting perspective (Duncan, 1992b).

Similarly, we believe that an approach that does not set a common factors context for change and validate the client's experience will not be salvaged by the most brilliant intervention. It is our assertion that the general considerations and the three criteria for designing competing experiences enables a useful balance between in and out-of- session opportunities for change.

Selection and Design: Case Example

Figure 5.1 depicts the factors involved in selecting and designing competing experiences. To illustrate this process-, rather than content-, oriented, series of decision points, the case of Eric, Terry, and Michelle will be examined in terms of the three general considerations and the multilevel description of change.

Dependence on the Client's Resources

Recall that this family presented with a suicidal adolescent requesting a second opinion regarding hospitalization. Although the new therapist began with the information that Michelle expressed suicidal ideation with a lethal plan (a friend had pills), and that a previous therapist had felt so strongly about the risk of suicide that he threatened the parents with child protection services if they did not comply with his recommendation for hospitalization, the new therapist did not begin

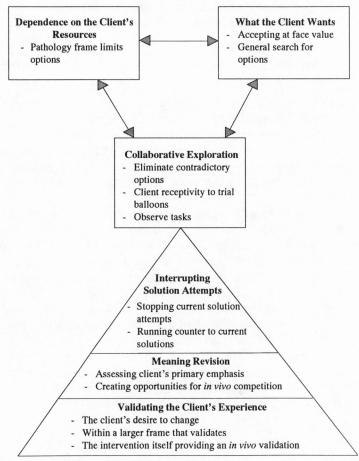

FIGURE 5.1. General considerations for selection and specific criteria for design of competing experiences.

therapy with a pathological frame of reference for Michelle or her parents. Not only did the therapist believe that this family had the resources necessary for problem resolution, but also he actively depended on the family having the inherent strength to overcome this suicidal crisis.

The recommendation for hospitalization and subsequent threat represented the antithesis to a view that seeks to utilize client strengths. The message was essentially, "You are incompetent to handle your daughter," which was offered with no opportunity for negotiation or even further discussion. The HMO therapist's lack of faith in the parents severely limited his solution alternatives and effectively destroyed any possibility for a working alliance. The new therapist began treatment with a recognized dependence on the clients' resources and found no evidence that suggested a shift to a less dependent position.

What the Client Wants

Recall that Eric and Terry wanted a second opinion regarding Michelle's suicide lethality and the recommendation for hospitalization. After their outrage was validated and their fears calmed by the negotiated no suicide contract, Terry brought up her ongoing conflict with Michelle and expressed a desire to get the therapist's input about that problem. Recall also that Michelle also identified the conflict with her mother as a problem and connected her mom's "harassment" to her suicidal inclinations.

The therapist accepted the clients' definition of the problem and the clients' goals for therapy. Eric and Terry's initial requests were directly addressed in the first session. Given that both Michelle and Terry identified ongoing conflict between them as a problem and both expressed a desire to address it, the focus and structure of the design process became the general problem description of parent–child conflict.

Accepting the problem of parent–child conflict at face value led the therapist to a consideration of several possible rationales and treatment options based upon previous experiences with parent–child conflicts and the clinical literature. Some intervention options were (1) conflict negotiation; (2) *quid pro quo* negotiation; (3) parent-effectiveness training; (4) behavior modification; and (5) giving up power, constructive payback.

Collaborative Exploration

At the end of the first interview, the therapist asked each family member to observe the conflict between Terry and Michelle, without intervention of any kind, so that they might obtain a naturalistic description of the conflict to share with the therapist in the next session. Given that the therapist had little information about the nature of parent–child conflict or any of the family's viewpoints, the observe suggestion was intended to enlist the family's help in the selection process by focusing their attention on the problem experience. It was also a possibility that such a suggestion might promote an opportunity for a revision in meaning about the problem, given that observing without intervention may represent an experience that competes with the family's current experience of the problem. A revision experience can be hoped for, but it can never be predicted in such situations.

Eric, Terry, and Michelle returned for session two, and the therapist began by separating the generations. Michelle went first. The therapist mentioned that he hadn't heard from Michelle, so he assumed that she wasn't thinking of killing herself. Michelle nodded and added that she didn't think it was a problem any more and that things were just piling up on her before. The therapist asked questions encouraging the elaboration of the current "no suicide" meaning system, and Michelle explained how things were much better. The therapist inquired about the observation task, and Michelle said that she didn't do it because she decided that she didn't want to work it out with her mother. Michelle reported that she just accepted that her mother was a bitch, and she wasn't going to let her mother get her down. Michelle wanted to discuss her boyfriend, and the therapist gladly obliged. The observe task resulted in Michelle bringing back new information about the problem and perhaps a revised meaning about her response to the conflicts, that is, they didn't bother her anymore.

Eric and Terry told a different story and described several incidents between Terry and Michelle that had escalated to screaming matches. Terry was unable to observe without intervention, which the therapist readily accepted as justified. At times, when Eric was away, Michelle would follow Terry around the house screaming obscenities at Terry at the top of her lungs. Terry was furious at Michelle and felt completely out of control. Although Eric witnessed several conflictual situations, Michelle seemed to always wait until Eric was out of town on business before escalating the conflict to extremes. The conflict nearly always arose from Terry's attempts to get Michelle to comply with household rules. Terry would remind Michelle several times, threaten her with consequences, and often attempt verbally to force Michelle to comply. Eric and Terry had grounded Michelle from the telephone, TV, and finally from everything. Nothing seemed to have an impact on the fights, and the extreme escalations seemed to happen more frequently. Even though Eric and Terry consistently enforced the rules and the consequences, the fights persisted. It seemed that Michelle, according to Eric and Terry, enjoyed the conflict and did her best to make everyone's life miserable, especially Terry's.

Additional exploration of Eric and Terry's idiosyncratic problem experience revealed that they both believed that Michelle was extremely manipulative, thoughtless, irresponsible, and selfish. Terry was very frustrated, given that she felt she had tried everything. Terry was a teacher and felt that she had thorough training in assertive discipline and behavior modification. Terry also felt powerless and was worried that Michelle was headed for disaster.

As the clients elaborated their experience of Michelle and Terry's conflict, their views of the problem and of Michelle, and what they had already tried, the therapist incorporated that input into an initial selection process and eliminated several possibilities. Given that Eric and

Terry perceived themselves as trying all forms of punishment and assertive discipline, the behavior modification and parent effectiveness training options were discarded.

The therapist introduced the idea of a form of negotiation between Michelle and her parents, and both Eric and Terry laughed at the prospect. Terry responded that until Michelle accepted responsibility around the house and gave Terry the respect she deserved, there could be no negotiation. Given the apparent contradiction to the clients' view, the intervention options of conflict negotiation and quid pro quo were discarded. Recall also that Michelle no longer wanted to work on the problem.

Eric and Terry provided a description of the problem experience that enabled the therapist to rule out choices that were already tried or were obviously contradictory to the clients' views. Eric and Terry also responded to ideas introduced by the therapist, and based on their receptivity, the therapist eliminated more options. The collaborative selection process led to the therapist's consideration of "giving up power to gain effectiveness" and "constructive payback" (Duncan, 1989; Duncan & Rock, 1991; Fisch et al., 1982).

Other aspects of Eric and Terry's presentation also indicated a good fit with the rationale for using these techniques. Eric, and especially Terry, were extremely angry and frustrated with Michelle and her behavioral antics. Both had exhausted direct attempts at influencing Michelle and, again, especially Terry, felt powerless and defeated, which only served to fuel her resentment toward Michelle. Such a problem scenario is quite congruent with the noted interventions, so the therapist decided to pursue a discussion with the clients to see if they too saw merit in the ideas. In addition to these general selection considerations, the multilevel description of change further specified the design of an individually tailored competing experience.

Interrupting Solution Attempts

Eric and Terry's solution attempts were characterized by direct efforts to obtain control over Michelle's behavior through coercion, exhortation, lecturing, confrontation, and punishment. The therapist asked himself two questions: What would stop the current solutions of Eric and Terry, and what other solutions would run counter to their current solutions? Giving up power and constructive payback were both ways of interrupting their solution attempts that were appreciably different from the current methods. "Giving up power" requires the verbal admission of powerlessness and entails making requests instead of demands. Constructive payback occurs when one person surreptitiously attaches a negative consequence to the irritating behavior of another person. Constructive payback can be helpful in giving parents some feeling of power and control and enables them to impose consequences for misbehavior (Fisch et al., 1982). The avoidance of the coercive and confrontive solutions may interrupt the problem cycle by undercutting the provocative and rebellion-inducing behavior that Eric and Terry were perhaps using. Different solutions employed by Eric and Terry may jam the coercion-screaming cycle and enable a new cycle of interaction to ensue.

Meaning Revision

Unfolding the conversation and exploration of the clients' experiences revealed that Eric and Terry were intensely angry at Michelle and tended to express only that aspect of their emotional reaction to Michelle's defiant behavior. They also felt powerless, hurt, and defeated.

Although Eric and Terry were asking the therapist for direct advice regarding what to do about Michelle's verbal abusiveness and irresponsibility, the therapist noted that the affective aspect of the problem experience was most salient. Given that the affective component was remarkable, the therapist sought to design the competing experience to target a contextual competition between the old affect of anger and a new affect of powerlessness, resignation, and inadequacy. The affectively altered problem experience could create an opportunity for a revised and perhaps more helpful meaning to evolve. Consequently, the therapist responded to Eric and Terry's request for direct advice and also suggested a competing meaning experience targeting an in vivo affective competition.

The therapist suggested that Terry give the following message to Michelle, as a way of giving up power to gain effectiveness:

"I have just talked to the therapist, and I realized a lot of things. You're right, I have been a bad mother. I should back off and leave you alone. I've been trying to control you and tell you what to do, and I can't. I always think I'm right and that I know what's best for you, and I don't. I am going to try my best to change, but you'll have to be patient with me. I've been this way for a long time. There will still be rules for you around the house, and consequences if you break them. But I realize it's up to you if you want to follow the rules, or put up with the consequences instead. I have finally accepted that your life is in your hands."

The therapist also suggested that Terry make requests of Michelle (not demands or threats) in the form of, "I would appreciate it if you would do the dishes. I know it's up to you and I can't make you do anything." Terry was encouraged to express the part of her that felt powerless and defeated, rather than angry, when she made such requests.

Terry liked the "giving up power" suggestion and commented on how it would enable her to take control of the situation while only giving in verbally. She also added that it only required her to admit something that had been apparent for some time: She really couldn't *make* Michelle do anything.

Constructive payback was introduced as a way of confusing Michelle and perhaps influencing her abusiveness, and as a way of discharging Terry's anger and frustration in a productive fashion.

TERRY: We are feeling abused and taken for granted on a daily basis. She really hurts me. She makes me feel out of control. I am at my wits' end.

ERIC: It really makes me mad. What should we do?

THERAPIST: I have an idea, but it's one that I am usually reluctant to offer, until I'm sure that two things are in the situation. The first is that the parents have to be real frustrated and even angry, because it takes a lot of effort to enact the suggestion.

TERRY: Oh we are . . . we both are.

ERIC: We're beyond frustration and anger; I'm ready to strangle the kid.

THERAPIST: Good! It takes that kind of determination. Second, it is a special tactic that is especially for the kid who is completely out of touch with other's feelings and is stuck in a way of perceiving the world that is thoughtless, disrespectful, and unconcerned about the effects of her behavior on others.

TERRY: That fits her to a tee. She isn't concerned with anyone or anything else but herself.

ERIC: Look, I'm ready to try anything. Michelle definitely has to change these abusive tirades.

THERAPIST: Well, O.K., I can see how your situation is one in which the tactic could apply—but I'm also hesitant to suggest this because it sounds so crazy that the benefits sometimes are hard to see. The tactic that is sometimes helpful to try is called constructive payback [Terry comments that she likes the name], and it is intended to shake her up and essentially turn the tables on her so that she becomes confused. She is perceiving you, Terry, in a disrespectful manner and needs to reorient her thinking. Through confusing her, she may shift her focus off of herself and onto the effects of her behavior on others. Let me stop here. Sometimes I ramble and don't make any sense.

TERRY: I understand what you're saying [looking intrigued], but how do we confuse her so she will have to reorganize her thinking? [Husband nods head in agreement.]

THERAPIST: Well, this is the crazy part. Constructive payback is the method of confusion. It entails paying her back shortly after she is abusive. In other words, it means that you pay her back for her inappropriate behavior—but for constructive purposes. For example, if Michelle yells at you or curses you, you may accidentally over- or undercook her food or put debris in her food [some laughter from both parents], or you may run the vacuum while she's on the telephone. It can really be anything that you know will be an annoyance to her, and it can take whatever creative and situation-specific form you can come up with. After you have constructively paid her back, and she confronts you with the evidence and inquires what in the hell is going on, it is quite important to this particular tactic to respond in a way that conveys a very humble apology and a sense of helplessness and hopelessness. In other words, things like, "I'm so sorry, I don't know what's gotten into me lately, I haven't been myself," "I must be losing my mind, how can I make it up. I've been depressed lately, and it must be affecting my mind," "I'm sorry, I feel so stupid," or anything in that vein. Basically, the position you want to convey is that you're terribly sorry and that you're either incompetent, stupid, senile, or crazy. It is often appropriate to be disgustingly sorry and self-effacing. Remember, I warned you that it's crazy. It is best if this strategy is presented from a position that looks like weakness instead of power, as we discussed earlier regarding giving up power to gain effectiveness. By not challenging Michelle for power, you can avoid a lot of the conflict and rebelliousness that would likely accompany more direct methods.

TERRY: It sounds great. I can get rid of a lot of hostility this way [laughing].

THERAPIST: Earlier I said that constructive payback requires a good bit of anger to implement, but it also is an effective and harmless method of discharging your anger in a way that may be helpful. It may allow you to channel that anger into doing irritating things back to Michelle, but in a planned way, designed to achieve a specific purpose. Finally, and judging by your laughter, you may feel the same way, it's all right to get a little secret enjoyment out of constructive payback.

Validating the Client's Experience

Giving up power and constructive payback were designed to interrupt the problem cycle of Michelle's abusiveness and Eric and Terry's confrontive solution attempts, and to create an opportunity for meaning revision through a suggestion that targeted an affective competition. The interventions were also designed to provide validation of Eric and Terry's experience of the problems with Michelle. The competing experience validated Eric and Terry's desire for change by directly addressing their goals of reestablishing parental control over Michelle's behavior, particularly her verbal abuse of Terry. Giving up power and constructive payback were delivered as part of a larger frame that validated their anger, frustration, and powerlessness. Consequently, Eric and Terry were in the position of experiencing the therapist's suggestions as between-session extensions of the validation context established in session. The competing experience itself provided an in vivo validation because it flowed from a perspective that was congruent with Eric and Terry's view that Michelle was acting inappropriately and in an inexcusably disrespectful manner.

Eric and Terry returned alone for session three, because Michelle had a gymnastics meet. Terry couldn't wait to tell the therapist about the ways she was able to pay back Michelle for her abusiveness and to share how much she enjoyed doing it to her! Terry reported that Michelle responded to powerless requests with great confusion—she often walked away shaking her head—and more important, she complied with the requests more frequently than ever before. On one occasion on which Terry refused to allow a friend of Michelle's to spend the night, Michelle became very loud and followed Terry around the house cursing her. Terry remained calm and did not respond to Michelle. Instead, she hung her head and mumbled to herself about where she had gone wrong with Michelle. Terry said she was able to stay calm by thinking of how she was going to pay Michelle back for the incident. The next day, Terry enacted constructive payback by "forgetting" to transfer Michelle's favorite outfit to the dryer, thereby delaying Michelle from meeting her friends at the mall. But that wasn't enough. When Michelle was finally ready to walk out the door, Terry stumbled and spilled a glass of milk on Michelle's blouse. Michelle was immediately furious, but Terry's rapid and pitiful apologies quickly turned her anger into confusion. Michelle told Terry that she was going seriously "weird" and that *she* was worried about *Terry*. Terry laughed and said to the therapist, "Mission accomplished."

Eric and Terry reported that they felt much better about Michelle and no longer felt burdened by her. They spent more time in couple's activities and less time discussing Michelle. Besides noting a more cooperative and less argumentative Michelle, Eric and Terry noticed a change in themselves. Before they felt inadequate and began blaming each other for Michelle's blowups. Now they felt in charge and were acting as a team to creatively handle Michelle differently. The therapist saw the family two more times. Michelle maintained that she did not feel suicidal. She broke up with her boyfriend and reported that she felt good about that. Michelle also added that things seemed better with her mother.

The therapist began treatment with a dependence on the inherent ability of this family to resolve its problems. The selection process evolved from the clients' desires and involved a collaborative give and take to determine a good fit. The therapist designed the competing experience to interdict the repetitive solution attempts, to create an opportunity for meaning revision, and to validate their experience of the problem.

DELIVERING COMPETING EXPERIENCES

In addition to the selection and design considerations, an important aspect of a competing experience is the style in which it is delivered or presented to an individual, couple, or family. Therapist style represents a way of interacting with clients that devalues the therapist as an expert and tends to be more cooperative, conversational, and relationship oriented. The style of delivery is not an independent factor but rather is directly linked to a conceptual framework for approaching clients and setting a common factors context for change. Therefore, the therapist's style of delivery is interwoven with both intervention and relationship factors. Three dimensions characterize a style that attempts to foster an atmosphere promoting common factors and client self-efficacy: (1) a *congruent* one down position (2) a collaborative stance and (3) an attitude of beneficent experimentation.

Congruent One Down Position

Success in therapy depends on, among other things, the ability of the therapist to engage the client in meaningful conversation and enlist the client's cooperation and expertise in dissolving the complaint that brought the client to therapy. Proponents of the MRI have advocated what they call "taking a one down" to elicit client cooperation in carrying out tasks or suggestions. The MRI asserts that although some people may respond well to authority or expertise, most people feel intimidated, demeaned, or embarrassed by a therapist position of one up and, therefore, will not share pertinent information or cooperate fully. Taking a one down or assuming a nonexpert role prevents the implication that the client has failed in seeing the appropriate solution already or that cooperation will be regarded as following orders (Fisch et al., 1982). The MRI emphasizes taking a one down as a tactic of persuasion that enhances both therapist maneuverability and client compliance.

As professional communicators, therapists need to develop a style that is both engaging and persuasive. Persuasive techniques, however, that are employed solely for effect, without a connection to the therapist's conceptual framework, may be perceived as patronizing or manipulative and undermine common-factor effects. If a therapist believes that he or she does really know the intricacies and complexities of human behavior and does have the solution or cure for the client, then taking a one down would be clearly incongruent and likely ineffective in fostering a cooperative environment.

We do not advocate the adoption of a one down solely for its effect, but rather because such a position genuinely reflects our theoretical orientation and assumptions about therapy. We advocate a *congruent* one down position because of a conceptual/pragmatic framework that discredits the belief in true maintainers or real causes of clients' problems.

Within this framework, the therapist is not an expert who champions an objective truth about the etiology and treatment of client problems or the way that life should be lived. Rather, the client is the expert from a perspective that places the client's meaning system and the client's input into the process in a hierarchically superior position to the therapist's orientation or input.

From an expert position, the therapeutic search is for interventions reflecting objective truths that promote change via the process of validating the therapist's theoretical point of view. The therapeutic search, from a congruent one down position, is for interventions reflecting subjective truths that promote change via the process of validating the client's meaning system.

A congruent one down position requires the humbling acceptance of the complexity of human beings and the utilization of qualifying language and tentative presentation when delivering competing experiences. Qualifying language consists of words such as "may" or "may not," "not sure," "seems like," "may be worth considering," etc. (Fisch et al., 1982); tentative presentation entails the genuine questioning by the therapist of the relevance and merit of the competing experience either directly by asking the client or indirectly through tone, facial expressions, and other nonverbals.

The therapist qualification and tentative presentation of the competing experience emerges from the therapist's belief that the intervention may or may not help and that it may or may not fit the client's perspective. Such a position of delivery not only conveys a nonexpert status, but also enhances client input into the process and gives clients the space to disagree with or modify the competing experience. A congruent one down position, therefore, helps foster a collaborative therapeutic relationship.

Collaborative Stance

Rather than being an expert armed with objective facts and powerful interventions, the therapist is a participant in a process in which opportunities for change are cocreated by virtue of the training and experience that the therapist brings and the resources, strengths, and personal expertise that the client brings. The therapist is a collaborator in co-constructing the conditions that will allow the client to resolve the problem that was the impetus for treatment.

Competing experiences are delivered in a way that conveys collaboration or working with the client or family as opposed to working on them. The therapist, by depathologizing problems, elevates the importance of the client's observations and perceptions and, therefore, enlists the client's help, participation, and collaboration when delivering a competing experience. A collaborative stance that values the client's resources and strengths contributes to a process that plants the seeds of self-efficacy that later grow and flower as clients empower themselves to resolve their own problems.

Just like empathy, respect, and genuineness, collaboration is a term that can be interpreted many ways by different clients, depending on their idiosyncratic life experiences, cultures, races, genders, etc. Similarly, the therapist needs to accommodate flexibly the collaborative needs of the client. For example, we are not suggesting that the therapist ought *never* to adopt a less collaborative stance. On the contrary, some clients may expect and even insist upon a more expert position and, therefore, will respond well to such a position. Just as some clients are not particularly interested in affective empathy, some clients will want direction from an authority in the field. In any event, it is the therapist who must flexibly adjust his or her behavior accordingly, based upon the client's presentation. Most clinical situations, however, seem more amenable to change when a collaborative atmosphere is fostered.

A congruent one down position devalues the expert role of the therapist and the therapist as a deliverer of truth. Such a position delivers competing experiences in a fashion that encourages client determination of the merit or relevance of the intervention and allows modifications of it. A congruent one down fosters cooperation and a collaborative context for change. A collaborative stance further enhances a delivery style that values client participation in the actual design and ownership of the competing experience. A collaborative stance paves the way for client self-efficacy by the therapist's reliance on the client's resources and input.

Beneficent Experimentation

Competing experiences are also delivered to the client with an accompanying attitude of beneficent experimentation. The therapist believes there are numerous possible interventions that could create opportunities for clients to resolve their problems and revise their meaning system. The therapist, then, delivers the intervention as a collaborator in a type of joint experimentation process. Beneficent experimentation overlaps considerably with a congruent one down and a collaborative stance, but also adds emphasis to both, as well as an added dimension. Beneficent experimentation not only conveys a nonexpert position and enhances collaboration, but also it implies that there are multiple solution alternatives with which to experiment.

Examples

"I have a couple of ideas that I would like to bounce off of you, but I'm not sure how on-target they are. Are you game?"

"This may or may not fit, but I was thinking that . . ."

"I wanted to ask you to consider an experiment that may help us learn more about your anxiety and how it may be improved."

"You know, therapy is not a definitive science, and I'm not sure what will help this situation. What I think may help is if we adopt an experimental attitude and try some things and then see if they help at all."

"I think I can suggest a few things, but I don't know whether they will fit your particular situation or will be helpful at all. This is where I need your help and wonder if you would be willing to try so and so and then let me know how it goes. Sometimes I may hit the mark, and other times I don't. How does that sound? Is it a good idea?"

"This may sound crazy, but I was thinking that it seems like your rituals are related to your relationship with your mother. Does that make sense?"

FOLLOW-THROUGH

Although the therapist and the client have a mutual understanding of the goals of therapy, and the therapist has selected, designed, and delivered the competing experience according to outlined criteria, competing experiences are not suggested with a specific meaning for the client to generate. Follow-ups related to between-session suggestions are, therefore, approached with a natural sense of curiosity and a desire for the client experience of intervention. Because there is no specific correct suggestion, the therapist continues the encouragement of input and remains prepared to amend, switch, or discontinue suggestions based upon that input. In other words, therapy is not a process of a client presenting a problem, the therapist conjuring up a definitive solution, and the client responding by miraculously being cured. Rather, therapy is a process of collaborative experimentation that remains flexibly open to feedback gained from the experimentation.

Unless the client has a more pressing concern, the therapist should inquire about the competing experience immediately in the next session. The therapist may ask the following questions: Did you get an opportunity to try what we talked about last time? How did it go? Did you notice any changes? Is that different than before? When a change is noted by the client, and perhaps a revised meaning has emerged, the therapist begins a series of questions designed to foster the elaboration and articulation of the change. This is called empowering client-ascribed meaning, which will be discussed in depth in the following chapter. Essentially, the therapist will strive to emphasize the role of the client in the change and deemphasize the role of the therapist.

Reported changes by the client may lead to termination or a decision to continue the competing experience or some modification of it. Recall Janice and her fear of flying. She returned following the symptom prescription reporting that her fears seemed more manageable. Based upon her feedback of her experience with the prescription and her newfound behavior of exploring what others thought and felt about flying, a new competing experience was designed. The airport rating task continued many aspects of the original prescription (different from avoidance, validation of her fears), but was modified as a result of the client's report of her experience.

Mark

Mark returned and reported that his concentration problem seemed to be related most to his lack of sleep. Exploration of the sleep problem revealed that Mark frequently woke up during the night worrying about school and getting his assignments completed. The therapist responded to the client's experience of the original observation task by suggesting another competing experience. The therapist again emphasized the significance of Mark's concern about school and the obvious importance of worrying about it, given how the worrying awakened him each night. The therapist asked Mark if he was willing to experiment with putting his worry to productive use in service of doing better in school. Mark nodded, and the therapist warned Mark that the suggestion was somewhat of an ordeal (Haley, 1984), and he may not want to try it and that was okay if he didn't. The therapist suggested that when Mark wakened during the night that he get out of bed and complete not less than 30 minutes of homework, even if he found himself drifting off to sleep during the 30 minutes. Mark returned and said that he was sleeping through the night, after getting up the first 2 nights and doing homework. Mark also reported that his concentration had improved significantly. In the cases of both Janice and Mark, the therapist constructed modified or different competing experiences based upon the feedback of the clients regarding their experience of the original interventions. Follow-through by the therapist requires the continued mutual exchange of ideas subsequent to a competing experience.

When There Is No Change

When the client reports that the competing experience did not lead to any changes or stimulate new information, the therapist explores how the suggestion was applied and what the client's perceptions are regarding the suggestion's lack of impact. The therapist pursues such information in a detailed fashion, as discussed in the initial interview chapter. The competing experience may have been agreed upon in the session, but when the client attempted to enact it, it somehow lost its relevance, or the client was unable to follow the suggestion for other reasons. No attribution of blame, pathology, or resistance is made by the therapist, and it is assumed that the client had good reasons not to enact the suggestion.

The reexamination of the competing experience may indicate that the therapist's perception of the goals need clarification and perhaps renegotiation. The very process of the client's thinking about the competing experience may have led to the client reevaluating the goals of therapy and consequently a different set of goals became more pressing. (Recall Michelle, who no longer wanted to work on her relationship with her mother.) Within this context of openness to client feedback and a genuine curiosity, a "failure" of an intervention becomes only a link in a larger chain of success.

Consider Donna, a 37-year-old secretary, who presented her problem as low self-esteem. The therapist suggested that she predict her level of self-esteem for the following day each night before retiring, compare the predicted level versus the actual the next night, and then attempt to make sense of the discrepancies if any existed. Donna returned and reported she had not attempted to follow the suggestion. Based on the assumption that, for whatever reason, the intervention was not a good fit, the therapist pursued what Donna's perceptions were of the suggestion. Donna said that the more she thought of her low self-esteem, the more she realized that her marriage was the biggest contributor to her lack of self-esteem. Donna's marriage became the new focus of therapy. The "failure" of the intervention led to new information presented by the client and a different goal for treatment.

Such occurrences are not uncommon and may result from between-session serendipitous events in the client's life that change the client's therapy needs or make the original suggestion lose its relevance. In the case of Donna, her husband went on a fishing trip, and she discovered that she didn't have low self-esteem while he was gone. Donna's situation is indicative of how clients often return with experiences that the therapist could not have expected. These unexpected responses by clients constitute perhaps the most enjoyable aspects of working with people. The flexibility of the therapist and his or her nonblaming openness to client feedback enhances the safety and security of the therapeutic relationship and sets the tone that encourages client confidence in risking new approaches to problems.

THE CASE OF JUDY

Judy, a 40-year-old female, was referred by her neurologist during inpatient rehabilitation. Judy was in rehabilitation after a cerebral vascular accident that affected extremities on her left side and bladder functioning. At the time of referral, Judy's physician reported that she was preoccupied with thoughts about cleanliness and was increasingly obsessed with using the commode. Attempts to reassure Judy that she was not dirty and did not need to use the commode so frequently were not working. In addition, Judy had just stopped taking medications for psychosis prior to her stroke, and the neurologist was concerned that Judy's behavior signaled the onset of another psychotic episode. The neurologist, who was reluctant to use antipsychotic medications in the early stages of stroke recovery, hoped that psychotherapy might help.

The initial interview with Judy included discussion with key staff persons (representing nursing, physical therapy, occupational therapy, and speech pathology). Through the interview process, the therapist learned that Judy and the staff's main concerns were centered around Judy's bladder retraining program.

This program was designed to address Judy's incontinence and urinary frequency. Nursing had begun by anticipating Judy's pattern of urination and transferring her to the commode before she urinated. This step had been successful, and Judy also made the next transition, which involved anticipating the need to urinate herself and calling the nurses for help. A snag occurred at the point that the staff was attempting to build Judy's bladder capacity. As a matter of standard procedure, this part of the program involved:

1. Encouraging Judy to hold her bladder after feeling the initial urge to urinate.
2. Encouraging Judy to increase time periods after the initial urge before calling the nurses for transfer to the commode.
3. Praising Judy for successfully increasing time periods without accidents.

In response to this plan, Judy had initial success. However, she also began asking questions about what would happen if she had an accident. Her concerns were addressed with reassurance to not worry about accidents. Staff reported that these reassurances did not seem to help and that over time Judy began to ask more and more questions about accidents. As reassurance became frustration on the part of staff, Judy began saying "funny" things about being unclean. In addition, rather than increasing periods of time between calls for transfer to the commode, Judy began making more frequent calls. As tension continued to mount, Judy had her first urinary accident, which exacerbated thoughts about being unclean, fears of incontinence, and calls to the nurses. At the time of referral, Judy was calling approximately once every five minutes.

During the initial interview, Judy spoke frequently about urinary incontinence and being dirty. She also defined dirtiness as a spiritual problem and asked the therapist if her priest could be brought to the rehabilitation center to give her absolution for her sins. She emphasized over and over that she would do anything to avoid another accident.

The therapist spent a great deal of time listening to Judy. The therapist acknowledged the emotional difficulty that naturally coincides with retraining a bladder that has done such a splendid job for so many years. The therapist expressed confusion about the connection between a urinary accident and the need for absolution. Claiming no expertise in this area, the therapist agreed to do what was possible to bring Judy's priest to the rehabilitation center. No attempts were made during this session to suggest a competing meaning experience, because Judy defined her problem as spiritual. Instead, arrangements were made with the attending physician's permission to honor Judy's request for a priest.

The therapist checked in with Judy shortly after the visit from her priest. She appeared more calm and relaxed, and expressed gratitude for being able to receive absolution for her sins. Despite this visit and receiving absolution, Judy still complained about not being able to stop the thought that she was unclean. When asked if she would like to work on this with the therapist, Judy agreed. The therapist proceeded with assisting Judy to specify attempts she had been making to stop thinking about being unclean. Attempts centered around giving herself messages to stop and telling herself that her thoughts were foolish. Dialogue related to solution attempts was followed by discussion about what would need to happen for Judy to know that she was beginning to improve. Judy stated, "I'd be less afraid of having accidents and would stop calling the nurses so much." The therapist delivered the following competing experience:

"From what you have said, the idea of urinary accidents is very troubling to you. This reaction is not surprising particularly given your age. After all, you are still young, and the idea of retraining your bladder at age 40 must be overwhelming.

I do have an assignment that might be worth experimenting with, for your unwanted thoughts, but before getting to that there is something else you might wish to consider.

Generally, in rehabilitation, and with cases like yours, accidents, though very unpleasant are actually considered to be critical steps in the right direction. You might even call them a necessary evil. Accidents mean you held your bladder too long, and, in your situation, for the long run, it is better to err by waiting too long than going too quickly. At least, that is what the doctors tell me.

Despite all that, these thoughts are still hard to shake, despite whatever reassurance I or others may give. Sometimes, though, in gaining control, the first step seems to be doing it on purpose. So, learning to stop these unwanted thoughts may mean at first seeing if you can make them happen. Would you be willing to try it?"

Judy replied affirmatively.

"You probably don't need to get too carried away with it, but, if for about 5–10 minutes a day or when you're waiting for therapy, see if you can make these thoughts happen. Then carefully observe the results and we can talk about it next week."

The therapist checked with Judy the following week and found her to be doing much better. She reported that she was no longer worrying about accidents and instead was thinking about whether she would need to apply for disability before leaving rehabilitation. (This was discussed, and arrangements were made with social services to pursue this matter further.) The nursing staff confirmed Judy's progress and stated that she was using the call buzzer much less. By the end of rehabilitation, Judy's bladder was successfully retrained. At the 1-year follow-up, she was continuing to adjust without remarkable difficulty.

Discussion

In this case, Judy's concerns and theories about change were placed in a hierarchically superior position to those of the therapist. No effort was made to counter the client's initial religious definition of the problem. The suggestion of a competing experience was withheld until it became part of a collaborative relationship with the client. The intervention was designed to block Judy's efforts at not having the thoughts by initiating an appreciably different solution of making the thoughts happen. The symptom prescription, therefore, was suggested to interrupt the problem cycle consisting of Judy's attempts to gain control over thoughts that seemed to happen involuntarily. Such a prescription offered a no-lose situation. If Judy could voluntarily make the thoughts happen, she would be taking the first step toward control. Future competing experiences would assist her with varying intensity levels or other aspects of the uncontrolled thoughts. Gradually, she could learn to stop them. On the flip side, failure to bring on uncontrolled thoughts deliberately would create a space where no such thoughts occurred. Future assignments could then involve increasing this space via this unusual form of failure.

Related to meaning revision, Judy's presentation reflected a strong emphasis on the cognitive aspects of the problem experience. Given the salience of a cognitive emphasis, the competing experience was designed to create a contextual competition between Judy's old ways of thinking about the problem (I can't control my thoughts) and new ways of thinking (make the thoughts happen; I am in control). Such a cognitively altered experience can enable the construction of an alternative meaning that provides a different solution alternative or renders the problem as no longer a problem. In Judy's case, the meaning simply emerged that the thoughts were no longer a problem.

The competing experience not only provided for the interruption of the problem cycle and enabled an opportunity for meaning revision, it also served as a vehicle to validate the client's meaning system regarding her unwanted thoughts. Judy received significant reinforcement from the staff to perceive her unwanted thoughts as unreasonable and, therefore, invalid. The staff's reassurance resulted in further frustration for Judy, which served as an impetus for Judy to try harder to gain control. Judy experienced her unwanted thoughts as out of her control, but at the same time, was encouraged not to worry about her bladder functioning. Judy also saw herself as foolish for having the thoughts. The intervention, therefore, was also designed to validate Judy's experience and legitimize her efforts at trying to control her unwanted thoughts. The prescription replaced the invalidation of Judy's and others' descriptions by highlighting their importance and legitimizing her concerns about her bladder functioning. The validation supported Judy in revising her meaning about the thoughts. It is interesting to note that Judy did not follow the prescription. The validation aspect alone perhaps provided all that was necessary for Judy to resolve her problem.

The assignment was delivered with a genuine sense of tentativeness. The therapist's intent was for Judy to accept the prescription willingly and not to view it as an imposition. Tentativeness deemphasized the therapist's position of authority and created a context in which Judy could have readily expressed reservations or refused the assignment. The client's right to reject the task was respected on the basis that the client is the ultimate authority on the problem and how it may be solved.

Judy thought about the suggestion, but did not enact the prescription, revised her meaning, and moved on to other problems before her next therapy session. The therapist expressed pleasure that Judy was feeling better, and the prescription was not reassigned. Because Judy no longer introduced uncontrolled thoughts, there was no need for the therapist to continue with that discussion. By allowing the client's presentation to determine the content of the therapeutic conversation, the problem of uncontrolled thoughts faded away as other topics emerged.

THE CASE OF LARRY

Larry, age 23, had been receiving community mental health services for 2 years. Bizarre thinking and behavior and an inability to maintain employment resulted in his placement in a socialization group for aftercare clients. Larry was also seen by the staff psychiatrist for medication.

Larry attended group regularly, and the main goal of treatment was keeping him stable enough to stay out of the hospital. This goal was successful; however, relationship problems between Larry and his father kept him on the edge. At home, Larry's mother tried to keep the peace and did so by expressing sympathy for both Larry and her husband. Her chief concern was her husband's threats to throw Larry out of the house if he did not find a job and stick to it. Larry's case manager observed that when family tensions were low, he complied with medications and did well in group. When tensions were high, Larry stopped his medications and became increasingly bizarre. The case manager's efforts to talk with Larry's father and help him understand Larry's condition had not been successful. He believed that Larry's main problem was irresponsibility, that is, refusal to clean his room, take care of his clothes, or find a job.

Larry's situation took a dramatic turn for the worse after Larry's mother was diagnosed as having a poor prognosis metastatic liver tumor. When Larry's mother failed to respond to chemotherapy, he became severely depressed and attempted suicide. Three psychiatric hospitalizations did not reduce Larry's suicidal thinking or attempts. While in the hospital, Larry would improve remarkably only to return to a state of depression shortly after discharge.

It was at this point that Larry, his father, and mother were asked by the case manager to come in for an interview with a therapist. The hope was that family problem solving might help Larry to stop his attempts at suicide and improve his adjustment to the impending death of his mother.

As the dialogue of the session unfolded, each family member addressed his or her most pressing concern. Larry's mother acknowledged that she had stopped all aggressive treatment for her cancer and was dying. Her last responsibility as she saw it was to insure that her husband and son reconciled. She felt that this was a critical concern, especially because of Larry's inability to fend for himself. Larry's father expressed anger that Larry refused to keep his room clean. He stated that he expected little and that the amount of debris and junk in Larry's room was beginning to overflow into the rest of the house. He was particularly upset because it seemed that while his wife was dying, Larry was sitting around, doing nothing, and scaring his mother with talk of suicide. Larry countered with the idea that he had tried to clean his room, but his efforts were not noticed. He also believed that his father did not understand the nature of his "chemical imbalance."

This conversation occurred with all three family members present. No separate interviews were conducted, because the mother had requested a family session, and both Larry and his dad expressed interest in a family problem-solving session. The therapist guided the interaction by seeking clarification, insuring that each member had the floor to speak, and by carefully legitimizing each person's position. At one point, Larry made a statement about his intent to clean his room that was so absurd that it made both parents, and especially his mother, laugh. The therapist highlighted this by praising Larry's ability to give his mother a good laugh during such difficult times. The following message and competing meaning experience was given:

"The first thing I would like to do is commend each of you for being here today. You are going through a time that is private, and I feel touched that you have been willing to share yourselves so openly with an outsider. I am also impressed with the amount of concern that you have as a family. Larry's ability to bring laughter to his mother, at a time of sadness and pain, is also quite impressive.

Because I am not you, I cannot know exactly what you are going through. Yet, a couple of years ago I lost my father to cancer and learned at a personal level about what it means to lose someone that you love. It was hard to watch him grow weaker and weaker and know there was nothing I could do. We also tried to carry out his last wishes.

It seems that as you have all described it, a major concern here today is Larry's relationship with his father. Mom, as I understand it, you want to see your men reconcile before you pass on. From what I can see, the men here want to work things out and their level of disappointment with one another shows how they are tuned into one another. When they don't think the other has given the right amount of love or respect, they become sensitive.

For this reason, I have a suggestion that you may wish to try. It may not help, but it is hoped that father and son might be able to explore some other dimensions of their relationship that might be worthwhile. Are you willing to do it? [The family agrees.]

During the coming week, Larry, your task is to secretly and without telling your father or mother, do something for your father that he would like. Dad, your job is to guess what that something is. However, the requirements of the assignment are for you to keep your guess secret until next week (O'Hanlon &

Weiner-Davis, 1989; Watzlawick et al., 1974). When we reconvene at that time, we will see what Larry did and find out if Dad guessed it. Mom, your job is to carefully observe your son and husband's relationship and look for changes in how they relate. Is the assignment clear?"

A week later the family reported that they had followed through on the assignment. Larry had taken a step toward cleaning his room. However, Dad especially noticed Larry making a greater effort to help him take care of his wife. Larry's mother reported that her husband and son seemed more relaxed together. Also, Larry did not threaten suicide and did not request psychiatric hospitalization. A few weeks later Larry's mother passed away. After 3 months, Larry was continuing to stay out of the hospital and was getting along better with his father. Larry still attended a socialization group and took medication. His group therapist was quite surprised when, after the death of a group member, Larry went out of his way to comfort another fellow group member who was grieving.

Discussion

In this case, the drama of the meanings centering around Larry's mother's death appeared to intensify the need for Larry and his father to address a long-standing problem in their relationship. This heightened intensity seemed to stimulate the interactional pattern of Larry's not meeting expectations to clean his room or find a job, and his father's expressions of disappointment. The interactional pattern was not understood as a function of a diagnosis, but rather as a reflection of unfortunate attempts at problem solving that were based on divergent meaning systems. Larry perceived himself to be victimized by a father who did not notice his efforts. His avoidance was based on the premise, "What's the use of trying?" Father, on the other hand, could find no evidence that Larry was trying to meet his expectations. Expressions of disappointment reflected an attempt to connect with Larry and obtain compliance.

This scenario of interaction seemed to create a context in which Larry and his father could not validate one another's position without acknowledging the incorrectness of their respective meaning systems, that is, father acknowledging his failure to notice Larry's efforts, Larry acknowledging his failure to follow through. This problem also occurred within the therapist–family relationship and suggested a critical dilemma. This dilemma involved finding a way to validate without disconfirming one or another family member's meaning systems. Disconfirmation could lead to a loss of rapport with one or another family member and undermine the therapist's ability to promote an opportunity that might lead toward change.

The competing experience interrupted the current solution attempts of all three family members by initiating behaviors appreciably different from Larry's avoidance of work, dad's expressions of disappointment, and mom's peacemaking role. The emphasis that Larry placed on the meaning of "being noticed" and the father's need to observe Larry "doing" provided useful information to the therapist for designing the homework assignment. The client-generated content suggested the direction of a behaviorally oriented competing experience. It was hoped that the experience of Larry being noticed and the father's observing Larry behaviorally meeting his expectations would create a new experience. This experience might allow father and son an opportunity to begin looking for the best in one another. Their behaviorally altered interaction with one another created an opportunity for meaning revision.

The experience of doing something nice and not telling, and observing and not telling was a way for the therapist to suggest such an experience, while simultaneously avoiding the pitfall of disconfirming father's, son's, or mother's meaning systems. The suggestion did not comment on who was right or wrong, but merely provided an opportunity for father and son to try something different. Not telling created a space where father and son could validate one another's experience without needing to admit the incorrectness of their positions. Mom's desire for reconciliation, Larry's desire to be noticed, and Dad's desire for Larry to take responsibility were all validated in the intervention. In the final analysis, the suggestion provided an opportunity for Larry, his mother, and his father to do the work and revise the meanings that best suited their needs.

Summary

This chapter has presented the selection, design, delivery, and follow-through of competing experiences. Competing experiences have been described as a widely ranging class of interventions that generally involve the therapist making a direct suggestion to the client in the form of a homework assignment in the hope of competing in some way with the client's actual experience of the presenting problem.

Competing experiences are action oriented and seek to alter the interaction surrounding the problem or the context in which the client's concern occurs. Although competing experiences target between session opportunities for clients to think, feel, or do something differently about the presenting problem, competing experiences also punctuate in session experiences and are based in criteria that emerge from the therapeutic conversation. Competing experiences are designed to interrupt the problem cycle, to focus on the most salient aspect of the problem experience, and to validate the client's desire for change and meaning system regarding the problem.

Competing experiences are often delivered from a congruent one down position to undercut the power disparity of the therapeutic relationship and to encourage clients to disagree with or modify the intervention. The therapist is a collaborator in a joint experimental process that seeks to create the conditions that will permit the client to resolve the presenting problem. Follow-through is approached with respectful curiosity with the therapist continuing to encourage client input and remaining open to modification, or discontinuing suggestions based upon the feedback from the client.

6 🪷 Revisions of Meaning

THE contextual competition promoted by competing experiences constructs the opportunity for an emergent meaning that either permits a different solution or is somehow less distressing. Competing experiences create the conditions for meaning revision and are *general* in focus, given that the attempt is to alter the context and not a preconceived or specifically targeted meaning. The interventions to be discussed in this chapter are specifically meaning focused and seek direct revision, replacement, or empowerment of a *particular* meaning system.

Because individuals continue to organize perceptions and make sense of their worlds apart from actual problem experience, acquired meaning systems can be revised via the ongoing dialogue of psychotherapy. Direct exploration of the client's perceptions and experiences of the presenting complaint may promote opportunities for the co-construction of alternative ascriptions of meaning.

Meaning emerges from ongoing interactions and is attached to memories of those interactions. Memories and their meanings are not static, but are constantly evolving recreations of past experiences (Rosenfield, 1988). Memory, therefore, is the recollection of the past in terms of present meaning. There is no recollection without a present context, and because interactive context is ever changing, there can never be a fixed absolute memory. It is the ongoing nature of meaning formation and the context-bound relativity of the memory process that makes meaning revision an ever-present possibility in psychotherapy.

Revision of meaning strategies are classified into two overlapping types that are differentiated from one another by the somewhat arbitrary distinction of who initiates the ascription of a different meaning. The two strategies are (1) empowering client-ascribed meaning and (2) therapist-ascribed meaning. Empowering client-ascribed meaning is an interventive process that requires the therapist to recognize a client shift in meaning, punctuate it, and encourage the elaboration and expansion of the new or revised meaning. Therapist-ascribed meaning represents the culmination of a meaning-revising conversation and offers an alternative meaning that permits different solution options or makes the problem less upsetting.

Throughout the process of psychotherapy, either during in-session exchanges of conversation or out-of-session client experiences, multiple possibilities for revision of meaning arise. In many ways, revision of meaning interventions are ones of opportunity. The therapeutic context inherently contains a reciprocity of these opportunities: Clients provide opportunities evolving from their enactment of competing experiences, serendipitous events, and the informal content of their presentations; therapists provide opportunities by suggesting competing experiences and the ascription of alternative meanings to the problem experience.

This chapter presents the clinical application of revision of meaning interventions. We discuss how the therapist can acknowledge and empower client ascriptions of meaning as well as elaborate guidelines for the therapist ascription of alternative meanings to client experience. This chapter also clarifies the role of insight in our approach and makes distinctions between client-ascribed meaning and insight, as well as among therapist-ascribed meaning, reframing, and interpretation.

INSIGHT AND CLIENT-ASCRIBED MEANING

The importance of insight in the change process of psychotherapy has been thoughtfully discussed and debated in the literature for many years. Those interested in the topic have been afforded innumerable opportunities to explore the pros and cons of one of the most, if not the most, polemic issues in our field.

Behaviorists were the first to challenge the assumption that insight is a necessary precondition for therapeutic change. Animal research demonstrating learning theory, and clinical research addressing the absence of symptom substitution in behaviorally oriented therapies, have been presented as arguments against the validity of the insight-leads-to-change causal link (Bandura, Blanchard, & Ritter, 1969; Masters & Johnson, 1970; Redd et al., 1979; Ullman & Krasner, 1975). Behavioral literature also documents that a change in behavior can lead to insight (Lazarus, 1971). The behavior research notwithstanding, adherents to insight-oriented therapies generally believe that therapeutic measures that do not uncover and resolve underlying conflicts or relate current problems to past determinants are thought to produce change that is precarious. The underlying belief of this position holds that the most disturbing sources of turmoil or the real cause of the problem will remain and eventually resurface in another form (Wachtel, 1977; Weiner, 1975).

Strategic theorists have taken a similar position to the behaviorists, and a review of the strategic literature reveals a significant amount of attention given to discrediting insight and the awareness–change link. Strategists typically view insight as unnecessary for therapeutic change and as a process that serves only to elongate therapy (Rohrbaugh & Eron, 1982). Haley, Madanes, and those associated with the MRI have asserted that (1) change is rarely accompanied by, let alone preceded by, insight; (2) insight or increased awareness sometimes occurs as an epiphenomenon or ex post facto rationalization after a change has taken place; and (3) looking for or exploring the causes of problems can actually prevent therapeutic change (Bodin, 1981; Haley, 1987; Madanes, 1981; Watzlawick et al., 1974). A strategic view of insight is probably best illustrated by the MRI statement, "In psychotherapy, it is the myth of knowing this 'why' as a precondition for change which defeats its own purpose" (Watzlawick et al., 1974, p. 87).

Both the traditional insight-oriented position and the anti-insight strategic and behavioral stance have outlasted their usefulness (Duncan & Solovey, 1989). Insight is not always a necessary precondition for change; many therapists observe change without insight and do not depreciate the significance of the change. On the other hand, insight is not merely an ex post facto rationalization, nor is its pursuit inherently self-defeating to psychotherapeutic change. On the contrary, insight and insightlike processes are invaluable phenomena that may be highlighted in therapy to enhance client change further. An alternative to the polemics described earlier is to accept that an insightlike process can and does occur, and then clarify its productive and efficient use in promoting rapid client change.

Client-Ascribed Meaning

Rather than one viewing insight as a prerequisite for change that must evolve from a long-term therapeutic encounter, or as an invariantly unnecessary impediment to change, insight may be understood in a context of meaning revision. A meaning revision context allows for the therapeutic facilitation of insightlike processes that significantly shorten the time typically believed to achieve insight. Competing experiences set the stage for these insightlike processes by promoting opportunities for meaning revision.

Following the suggestion of a competing experience, clients often return to report enhanced self-awareness and increased knowledge about the problem that has apparently emerged from events that occurred between sessions. These client reports bear a striking resemblance to what many therapists would call insight, even though the process by which the insight was achieved could not be adequately explained by traditional insight approaches.

From a meaning revision perspective, these insightlike client reports are indications that the client has experienced a shift in meaning and has ascribed a new or revised meaning to him- or herself or the problem experience. These *client-ascribed meanings* represent a culmination of a meaning revision process that evolves from the client's attempts to enact, or actual enactment of a suggested competing experience. New meanings also arise from serendipitous events or other outside of therapy experiences unrelated to in-session conversations.

Recall the cases of Mark, Mary, and Janice from Chapter 5. In each case, the therapist suggested a competing experience that provided an opportunity for meaning revision. Through the clients' enactments of those competing experiences, new and revised meanings were ascribed by the clients. Mark revised his meaning regarding his concentration problem to include a connection between his lack of sleep and his ability to concentrate. Exploring and expanding Mark's ascribed meaning led to different and effective solutions to his concentration problem.

Mary attributed the meaning of "being too reliant" on her marriage to her previous behavior regarding her husband. Her newly ascribed meaning enabled Mary to broaden her social network and independently pursue her own happiness. Janice returned and reported that her fears were more manageable and that she had discussed flying with others. The therapist viewed Janice's new insights as an indication that a meaning revision occurred and explored other ways of expanding and reinforcing Janice's newly ascribed meanings.

Serendipitous events also stimulate a context for meaning revision. Recall Donna and her low self-esteem. Donna chose not to act on the suggested competing experience, but an unexpected event facilitated the emergence of a revised meaning that she reported in the following session. Donna's husband went on a fishing trip, and she learned that she did not have low self-esteem while he was gone. His absence fortuitously created a context for Donna to ascribe a new meaning to her low self-esteem that related it to her relationship with her husband. The client-ascribed meaning led to renegotiation of the therapeutic contract and the emergence of different solution options.

Regardless of how a new client ascribed meaning may be precipitated, the fact that clients bring back revised meanings to the therapeutic conversation is a testament to both the ongoing nature of meaning formation and the client's inherent ability to resolve the presenting problem. Experiencing these insightlike phenomena with clients has led to a conceptual comparison between insight and client-ascribed meaning, and ultimately to an intervention process designed to seize the opportunities for continued change that client-ascribed meanings represent.

Insight versus Client-Ascribed Meaning

Insight, in the traditional dynamic sense, can be defined as the conscious experience, integration, and modification of unconscious conflicts and past influences so that a change occurs in the person's general framework, enabling a reorganization of information processing and the belief about oneself (Weiner, 1975). Insight, in a generic and simplified sense, may be considered a process in psychotherapy wherein psychological and familial problems are altered via increased knowledge concerning the determinants of the problem and/or awareness of self.

Two distinctions may help clarify the difference between client-ascribed meaning and insight (Duncan & Solovey, 1989). Insight occurs as the result of the gradual accumulation of many interpretations by the therapist. Over time, the therapist builds his or her case, carefully selecting interpretations on the basis of depth, focus, timing, and connotation. The therapist, therefore, generates or promotes the insight based upon the invariant content of his or her theoretical orientation.

Client-ascribed meaning, on the other hand, is client generated, as opposed to therapist generated. Clients are offered competing experiences that enable the opportunities for meaning revision. Competing experiences are presented to the client in the spirit of collaborative experimentation such that the message is conveyed that something of value may happen, and the client should pay close attention to the situation under concern. No particular meaning is targeted, and the therapist has no specific meaning in mind. Given the general and sometimes abstract nature of many competing experiences, clients are presented with situations in which they not only must construct meaning about the tasks involved, but also about what the competing experiences mean when applied in their social contexts.

The competing experience is a general framework for meaning revision that clients idiosyncratically apply to their problematic situations and then independently formulate specific, non-therapy-originated meanings. The intervention can be thought of as an abstract and general outline of an experience through which the client fills in the concrete and specific details of particular ascribed meanings. Client-ascribed meanings seem to occur spontaneously in response to attempts to enact, or actual enactments, of general suggestions that start the change process in motion. These client-generated, independently formed revised meanings often lead to solutions that reinforce the new meanings and vice versa.

Insight-oriented approaches tend to view insight as a necessary precondition for change and believe that change occurring without insight is spurious or short-lived. Client-ascribed meaning, conversely, occurs during the process of change or when the client is thinking, feeling, or doing something different regarding the presenting problem. Client-ascribed meaning may also occur as a postcondition of change as clients organize their perceptions about their altered experience of the presenting problem.

The two distinctions (insight is therapist generated and emanates from a particular theoretical frame of reference, client-ascribed meaning is client generated; insight is a precondition of change, client-ascribed meaning occurs during change or afterwards) permitted the consideration of how the process of client-ascribed meaning could be enhanced and further empowered in psychotherapy (Duncan & Solovey, 1989). The more sensitive we become to a client's reports of new information about the problem and increased self-awareness, the more impressed we become with the value of placing the client's newly ascribed meanings in a primary position in the therapeutic plan. These new meanings are important opportunities for intervention that potentially could result in rapid problem resolution.

Recall from Chapter 1 the research concerning the factors that contribute to positive outcome in psychotherapy. Accounting for as much as 40% of the outcome variance are so-called spontaneous remission variables such as out-of-therapy events and other client-specific variables (Lambert, 1986). Remission (improvement) from our perspective may not be truly spontaneous, but rather a *probable* result of the inevitable responsiveness to variation provided by the therapy experience and the meaning-revision context it promotes. Client responses to competing experiences and other idiosyncratic and serendipitous events occurring between sessions create invaluable opportunities for the therapist to enhance the powerful spontaneous remission effects. Spontaneous remission variables are therefore *expected*, given the therapist's belief in the ongoing nature of meaning revision, the inherent resources of the client, and the explicit context for meaning revision that psychotherapy provides.

Spontaneous remission is perhaps facilitated by competing experiences and therapist openness to utilize spontaneous remission effects (i.e., new meanings) that clients identify as significant to their improvement, whether directly or indirectly related to in-therapy events. This facilitation process is the essence of empowering client-ascribed meaning.

Empowering Client-Ascribed Meaning

The potentially rapid facilitation of an insightlike process and the enhancement of the powerful effects of spontaneous remission variables represent compelling reasons to place the client's presentation in a hierarchically superior position to the therapist's orientation. Empowering client-ascribed meaning is an intervention process or sequence that requires the therapist to *trust* in the probability of meaning revision, to *recognize* when a shift in meaning has occurred, and then to *promote* a conversational context that unfolds and expands the new meaning.

It is important that the therapist trust in the process of client-ascribed meaning and the inherent abilities that the client possesses to resolve problems. Many therapists make clinical assumptions guided by the content of their theoretical orientations that result in missed opportunities to utilize clients' ascriptions of meaning. Placing the content of the client's presentation before the therapist's agenda allows the therapist to be attentive to opportunities when they emerge. To trust the process is to trust that the client's presentation, both initially and during all phases of treatment, will provide opportunities for rapid meaningful change.

Recognizing New Meaning

Recognition of a shift in meaning requires a childlike curiosity in a therapist who is expecting an inevitable revision in meaning or change each time the client returns. As discussed in Chapter 5, subsequent to the suggestion of a competing experience, the therapist follows up by inquiring about the client's experience of intervention. If no intervention was suggested, then the therapist inquires about any changes in the problem or in the client's circumstance since the last visit that the client would like to tell the therapist. This openness to client feedback not only conveys the collaborative nature of the relationship, but also enables the therapist to attend to any indications that a meaning shift has occurred. Indications include client presentation of new information, heightened self-awareness, improvement of the presenting problem, a change in affect, and/or changes in physical appearance or even seating arrangement. This is not to say that every time a therapist notices a difference in seating arrangement, or any other possible indicator, that a shift has actually occurred. Rather, such indications do signal the possibility of a meaning shift that the therapist should pursue to see if, indeed, there has been any change.

Consider Carol and John, who entered therapy because John had lost desire for sex, and because a general malaise characterized their relationship. After the first session, which validated both Carol and John's experience of the marriage, the therapist asked the couple to note the things they observed in the marriage they would like to see continue (a formula task of de Shazer, 1985). Carol and John returned for session two, and the therapist immediately followed up on the competing experience. Both reported several things they noted, and both observed a decrease in overall tension. The therapist responded with amazement, pleasure, and a natural curiosity about what was going on with the couple. The therapist observed that something else seemed different—the couple was laughing and sitting close to each other—and asked the couple if that meant anything. Carol giggled and replied that John had suddenly become romantic. John didn't know what happened, except that he had suddenly felt full of desire.

The therapist recognized several indications that a shift in meaning had occurred and pursued it. Pursuing these indications revealed that the couple had spontaneously resolved the very problem that had brought them to therapy.

Promoting New Meanings

Once clients report new perceptions regarding themselves or their problems as a response to either competing experiences or serendipitous events, and the therapist has recognized the report as a shift in meaning, then the therapeutic focus becomes a promotion of a therapeutic dialogue that will expand and further empower the new meanings created by the clients. Through questions that encourage the client to articulate and embellish the reasons behind the changes of circumstances or heart, the therapist amplifies the change that has transpired. Further change is empowered through the client's own positive ascriptions without the therapist taking responsibility for the change or assuming a cheerleader role. Therapeutic movement is thus further amplified as the therapist encourages the client to expand the meaning and continue progress regarding the presenting complaint. Clients gain momentum for change by describing the changes they have experienced and essentially get on a roll of positive self-ascriptions.

Examples of questions that encourage clients' further articulation of client-ascribed meaning include:

How were you able to do that?
What brought you to that conclusion?
That's great—but I'm not sure how you arrived at . . . (particular situation, meaning, or solution)
To what do you attribute this turn of events?
I'm confused, what does all this mean?
Why did you decide to . . . ?
How were you able to overcome the temptation to . . . ?
This is different, what is going on?
Can you fill me in on what led you to . . . ?
This is an amazing turn of events—but I'm puzzled, help me understand how this could have happened.

Empowering client-ascribed meaning seizes opportune shifts in meaning and fosters an environment that promotes the continued ascription of meaning of the client. The therapist can actually observe meaning formation in action as the client organizes perception and experience to articulate answers to the meaning-expanding questions of the therapist.

Case Examples

Alice and David

Alice and David sought therapy for their 13-year-old daughter, Jill, who had superficially cut her wrist after an argument with her parents. On another occasion, Jill had threatened to kill herself. The parents were very concerned and described Jill as an overemotional child who was very different from her two older sisters. Jill's sisters were academically successful, attractive, and quite popular. Alice and David were most troubled by the suicide threat, but also identified Jill's emotional outbursts as important as well. David was particularly concerned about the long-term consequences of Jill's inability to control her emotions. The therapist interviewed the family together and also interviewed Jill and her parents separately to permit the explicit validation of each person's meaning system. At the end of the first session, to all three family members, a competing experience in the form of a formula task was suggested. The parents were asked to observe Jill closely and note the things they observed that they would like to see continue (de Shazer, 1985).

The family returned in 3 weeks and responded to the question of what they had observed with a long list of positive events and attributes. Jill was perceived as more communicative, more cooperative, and able to keep her emotions in check. The therapist responded to each item on both parents' lists with follow-up questions that encouraged further articulation. For example, when David said that Jill was able to control her emotions, the therapist asked him if he could give specific instances that precipitated the observation. The therapist believed there was more meaning revision to be encouraged and pursued a sequence of questions with Jill's parents alone.

David reported that he had gotten in the habit of looking for the bad in Jill and that he was quite critical of her. Looking for the good in her allowed him to notice that she was a pretty neat kid and that she had strengths that Jill's two older sisters did not have. The therapist continued to pursue by asking follow-up questions like, "What strengths are you referring to?" David continued and said that he felt his relationship with Jill was also better, and he was able to back off his critical style. He said that he found that he liked himself better as a parent and felt better about his relationship with Jill. The therapist asked for further clarification, and

David concluded that he was most pleased with his own changes in parenting style.

This case illustrates the use of client-ascribed meaning to empower and encourage change. A competing experience was suggested that created an opportunity for meaning revision; no particular meaning was intended. Alice and David gave meaning to the task, and a variety of new meanings were ascribed in their application of the task. Note that David decided to "back off" and seemed more concerned about his relationship with his daughter, as opposed to his previous presentation. There had been no prior discussion of either issue, and the therapist did not suggest any changes regarding parenting style. The meaning that evolved and the resulting changes (backing off, appreciating strengths, feeling better about self as a parent) were formed independent of the therapist. Once the therapist recognized the changes, the task was one of empowerment; the therapeutic work was essentially done. Jill also ascribed a new meaning when she reported that she found that she could get more out of her parents if she didn't blow up at them. The case was terminated in the second session.

Monte

Monte sought therapy because he feared he was going crazy. Monte's father, who had died when Monte was a small child, was schizophrenic. Monte noticed an increase in his overall level of anxiety about 5 years previously, which escalated to the point where he had experienced high levels of anxiety every day for the prior 2 years. On many occasions Monte experienced panic attacks, which he characterized as the worst times of his life. Monte's greatest fear was that he would wind up like his father, hopelessly mentally ill in an institution.

A variety of different opportunities were pursued by the therapist (e.g., relaxation training, observation tasks, the meaning of the anxiety, etc.), both in and out of session, but none of the options explored or enacted had any impact on Monte's anxiety. In the fourth session, the therapist directed focus back to the specifics of the problem, hoping to find more opportunities. Monte said that he realized he was going to have a bad day immediately after awakening. The therapist suggested a competing experience in the form of a symptom prescription, which was suggested as an experiment to see if anything else occurred to Monte in the throes of an actual panic attack. Monte was asked to bring the anxiety on as intensely as he could immediately after waking and determining that he was going to have a bad day.

In the next session, the therapist asked Monte how the experiment had gone. Monte replied that he hadn't had a bad day since he last saw the therapist 2 weeks previously. Because he did not have a bad day, he didn't bring on the anxiety. The therapist began a series of questions intended to flesh out the details of this surprising turn and to encourage Monte to ascribe self-empowering meaning to the noted changes. Monte reported that he felt so good that he had quit smoking 2 days after his last appointment and that he felt like he had taken control over his life. The therapist was genuinely awestruck! Not only had Monte felt free of anxiety, but had tackled the very difficult, anxiety-producing task of stopping smoking.

Monte was amused by the therapist's amazement and added that being able to quit smoking was the kick in the butt he needed to boost his self-confidence. Monte returned for the final session 1 month later. Monte maintained both major gains; he no longer felt uncomfortably anxious or experienced attacks; and he still was not smoking. Monte added that for the first time in 2 years, he did not dread getting out of bed each day. The therapist continued to ask questions designed to promote further empowerment of Monte's self-confidence. The conversation ended with Monte saying that although he couldn't really explain why he felt so much better, it seemed that quitting smoking helped him realize that he could make things better and that he could take control over his life.

The therapist could not have predicted that Monte would quit smoking and that such an experience would provide Monte with a new meaning of self-confidence and control. It is unknown what role the symptom prescription played, and in many ways it is irrelevant. What is relevant is that an opportunity arose from a serendipitous action by the client that enabled a new meaning to be ascribed. The therapist took the opportunity and promoted a conversational context that allowed Monte to continue to ascribe meaning to his actions and; thus, be further empowered by his own words and positive self-ascriptions.

Empowering client ascribed meaning, in its essence, is a fundamen-tally growth-enhancing intervention that pursues a client-reported change and punctuates it, expands it, and generalizes it to include as much affirmation to the client as possible—and all in the client's own words.

THERAPIST-ASCRIBED MEANING

The therapist ascription of alternative meaning to the client's problem experience is more commonly referred to in the literature as *reframing*. Since Gregory Bateson (1955) coined the word *frame* to describe the organization of interactional patterns, many have utilized that description to develop interventions that reorganize or reframe problem behavior in the context of psychotherapy. To reframe, as classically defined by the MRI, is "to change the conceptual and/or emotional setting or viewpoint in relation to which a situation is experienced and to place it in another frame that fits the facts of the same concrete situation equally well or even better, and thereby change its entire meaning" (Watzlawick et al., 1974, p. 95).

There are a wide variety of ways to reframe client circumstances that are documented in the literature, ranging from simple relabeling (e.g., referring to depression as realistic pessimism), to positive connotation (e.g., referring to the bizarre behavior of a schizophrenic as creative ways of meeting the individual's needs or as altruistically motivated to stabilize the family system), to redefining (e.g., referring to adolescent rebellion as necessary steps toward individuation). Reframing essentially attempts to initiate a difference in the client's current "frame" regarding the problem in the hope of reconstructing it in such a way that makes remedial action possible or renders the problem no longer distressful. Consider the following examples and the different ways in which an alternative frame of the client's experience was presented by the therapist.

Recall Anita from Chapter 2, who was hospitalized following a suicide attempt and was subsequently diagnosed with BPD. The diagnosis became an inhibitor to the client's taking action to help herself feel better, as well as a justification for her husband to ignore her legitimate concerns about their relationship. The therapist asked Anita, "What if you are not a BPD," and later suggested that a different diagnosis (one less debilitating) might be more accurate. Anita, no longer enslaved by the implications of her diagnosis, addressed her marital problems and sought fulfillment outside of her mother/wife roles. Reframing was in the form of a question and then involved a relabeling of Anita's experience; the frame was largely cognitive in focus.

Sue's husband Johnny had intended to kill her and himself when he received the divorce papers in the mail. He called Sue and said that he was upset over being separated from his 3-year-old son. When Sue refused to meet him, he made sure she was listening over the phone and shot himself in the head. Johnny's parents blamed Sue and sued her for the meager estate to recoup the cost of burying their son. Sue blamed herself for Johnny's suicide, even though her decision to divorce him was because of his cocaine addiction and his inability to hold a job. She started using pot and neglecting her son. When she told the therapist about the way Johnny killed himself, the therapist responded angrily, pounding his hand on the desk, calling Johnny a son of a bitch for doing that to her. Shocked at the therapist's outburst, Sue asked what he meant. The therapist replied that it was unfair that she be blamed for saving her own life and making a decision to survive as a parent for her son. This was the first recognition of Johnny's involving her in the suicide to hurt her and how unfair this was to her. Sue took the first steps to getting her life in order and becoming a responsible parent once again. The therapist reframed Sue's guilt and depressive emotional response to Johnny's suicide through his angry emotional reaction to her description of the suicide. The changed emotional context (guilt to anger) enabled Sue to address her parenting responsibilities with the therapist and to begin attending Narcotics Anonymous (NA) meetings.

Doris, a 41-year-old nurse, presented her problem as depression, largely revolving around her guilt and shame about an incestuous relationship she had had with her stepfather at age 16. Doris perceived herself as a willing and active participant in the incest, and she felt particularly distressed when she remembered that she enjoyed the sex, as well as the step-father's company. Doris felt she not only was a degenerate for enjoying the sex and remembering it with excitement at times, but also the worst kind of person to betray her own mother in that way.

After a discussion about the power discrepancy between a 40-year-old "man of the world" and a 16-year-old virgin, naive girl, the therapist asked the client how she would view the following scenario. The therapist described a situation in which he (the therapist, who was approximately the age of her stepfather) went into a fast food restaurant and encountered Doris's 16-year-old daughter working behind the counter. The restaurant wasn't busy, so the therapist stayed and chatted with the young woman using his 20-plus years of experience at seduction. Her daughter, becoming somewhat charmed by the smooth style of the older man and feeling pleased by the attention, impulsively agrees to meet the man after work.

The therapist stopped and asked Doris what she was thinking. A discussion ensued that emphasized not only the discrepancy of life experiences, but also the premeditated intent by the older man to manipulate the 16-year-old to achieve his own sexual satisfaction. The reframing occurred in the form of the scenario presented by the therapist that allowed Doris to experience her relationship with her stepfather in a different conceptual context, that is, from a view that she was an active and equal participant to a view inclusive of the gross inequity of her experience with her stepfather. The problem of guilt and shame was rendered no longer a problem.

In each example, a different frame for the client's experience was offered by the therapist using a variety of formats (questions, an emotional response, and an imaginary story). Each format reframed the problem context in such a way that accomplished a shift in client perspective so that the problem became solvable or no longer distressing.

Therapist-Ascribed Meaning versus Reframing

While the previous cases illustrate reframing, they also exemplify an expansion of it that we call therapist-ascribed meaning. This expansion largely refers to a consideration of the interdependence of technique and relationship. Discussions in the literature describe the "technique" of reframing but do little to explain how reframing fits in the context of the therapeutic alliance. While reframing constitutes a large part of therapist-ascribed meaning, the former is extended by three additional conceptual and practical features: (1) therapist-ascribed meaning represents the culmination or punctuation of a collaborative process between the client and therapist; (2) therapist-ascribed meaning is an explicit therapist behavior that both validates the client's experience *and* offers an alternative perspective; and (3) therapist-ascribed meaning utilizes frames or meanings from any possible source, including other therapy approaches.

The therapist ascription of an alternative meaning to the problem, solutions, and/or context of the presenting complaint represents the culmination of a process between the client and therapist. Therapist-ascribed meaning emerges from a free exchange of ideas and meanings that allows an ever-present opportunity for the client to reexperience his or her problem situation. Through this mutual search of the client's content-rich presentation, other descriptions, implications, connections, and distinctions may evolve. Rather than representing a unilateral technique formulated by the therapist to change the client's experience of the problem, therapist-ascribed meaning is reflective of an ongoing conversational context that promotes the construction of alternative meanings by the client or the therapist. The therapist merely highlights the emergent meaning or the meaning exploration process itself by offering an alternative perspective for the client to consider.

The therapist's questioning of the accuracy of the BPD diagnosis of Anita occurred after a discussion of how her BPD restricted her and absolved her husband of responsibility to address Anita's marital concerns. A flavor of questioning the validity of her diagnosis characterized the conversation. The therapist-ascribed meaning simply emphasized what was already happening.

Recall Sandra from Chapter 4 and her presentation of a depression that fell on her out of the blue. Exploration of Sandra's perceptions and experiences associated with the depression enabled her previously unstated connection between her husband's impotence and her depression. Through the unfolding of her experience, Sandra created a new meaning for her depression and no longer viewed it as occurring for no reason. Flowing from that newly emerged meaning, the connection between the depression and the impotence was punctuated via a therapist-ascribed meaning.

The connection the client had already made was further amplified by the use of a meaning, emanating from a Milan family therapy perspective, called "positive connotation" (Selvini-Palazzoli et al., 1978). The therapist suggested that perhaps both her depression and her husband's impotence functioned to protect the marriage from conflict or divorce. If it were not for Sandra's depression, she might think enough of herself to find a partner capable of providing the sexual intimacy she desired, and if it were not for her husband's impotence, he might grow tired of living in a relationship with a depressed person. So in a strange kind of way, the depression and the impotence held the marriage together. Sandra replied by suggesting that both problems were like the glue holding everything together.

Rather than a frame magically and unilaterally designed by the therapist, the therapist-ascribed meaning connecting the client's depression to her husband's impotence emerged from the mutual exploration of Sandra's presenting problem. The therapist-ascribed meaning evolved from a collaborative description of the problem, pulled together several elements of the client's presentation (her depression, his impotence, his previous affair, etc.), and offered yet another way of viewing her depression as related to her marriage. Given that therapist-ascribed meaning is co-constructed from the interactional process, it is more collaborative than reframing. The new meaning is therefore not imposed, but rather cogenerated.

Just as competing experiences offer an opportunity for the therapist to explicitly demonstrate empathy, respect, genuineness, and validation of the client's experience, therapist-ascribed meaning simultaneously respects and validates the client's experience while offering an alternative perspective. Recall Sue and the blame she received from others and herself regarding Johnny's suicide. Her own view contained significant invalidation of her experience, as evidenced by her questioning her decision to divorce Johnny and the responsibility she accepted for his death. The therapist-ascribed meaning replaced that invalidation with the therapist's response of indignation to Johnny's suicide. Not only was the suicide a terribly traumatic event in and of itself, but it also was an incredibly horrendous thing for Johnny to do to her. Sue felt that she had done the right thing for the first time in the 9 months following Johnny's death. The therapist-ascribed meaning validated her experience, in addition to offering a different perspective.

Similarly, Sandra's initial presentation also contained invalidation of her experience, given Sandra's perception that there was no reason for her depression. ("I should be happy.") The conversation progressed to the point that the client replaced her own invalidation with a connection of her depression to her unsatisfactory relationship with her husband. The therapist-ascribed meaning (positive connotation) further validated that connection while suggesting an alternative view.

Finally, therapist-ascribed meaning extends the technique of reframing through its access to meanings from other therapy approaches. Strategic views have long discredited insight-oriented approaches and have ignored the rich source of meanings they provide. Therapist-ascribed meaning embraces different and seemingly antithetical approaches as providing a multitude of different meanings that the therapist can respectfully add to the therapeutic process. Rather than viewing psychoanalytic, structural, or any other approaches as being incorrect, utilizing therapist-ascribed meaning requires the acceptance of each view as one view among many that may provide a meaning for the client's experience that is both validating and helpful. This openness to a variety of available meanings allows for a flexibility that is focused not on a single orientation, but rather on the emergent process in session, the client's content presentation, and the degree to which one particular theoretical orientation "fits."

Therapist-Ascribed Meaning and Interpretation

Therapist-ascribed meaning sometimes looks like what insight-oriented therapists call interpretation. Interpretation can be defined as "a statement that refers to something the patient has said or done in such a way as to identify features of his behavior that he has not been fully aware of" (Weiner, 1975, p. 115). Interpretation is intended to expand clients' awareness of their thoughts and feelings and thereby enhance their understanding of themselves (Weiner, 1975).

There are two major differences between therapist-ascribed meaning and interpretation. Interpretation offers clients a way of looking at their dilemma that is based upon the therapist's frame of reference or theoretical orientation. A psychodynamic therapist may interpret unresolved conflict, a cognitive therapist may interpret irrational and self-defeating thoughts, a transactional analysis therapist may interpret client games and ego states, and a transgenerational family therapist may interpret the family ledger or legacy. Implicit in the notion of interpretation is its representation as a more accurate way for clients to perceive their problems.

Therapist-ascribed meaning is not intended to offer a better way of understanding the client problem, or a true meaning of the situation, because the ascribed meaning is not based on the adherence of the therapist to any particular orientation. We are, therefore, interested in pursuing alternative meanings to problem situations rather than correct or true meanings. No inherently correct meaning is pursued because of a belief that there is no "true maintainer" of the presenting problem, that is, there are no specific preconceived ideas that account for problematic behavior (e.g., oral fixation, confused hierarchy). Recall from Chapter 2 that this is a "process" view that asserts no particular "content" as an explanatory scheme for client problems (Held, 1986). Change occurs through interactive process and meaning revision, rather than through the pursuit of a particular content.

Because no particular theoretical or content path must always be followed, the therapist may ascribe many different meanings to problem situations. The therapist is, therefore, free to select and offer "true" meanings from any approach that seems to fit the client's predicament and that validate the client's experience.

Recall Sandra and the therapist-ascribed meaning that emphasized the connection of her depression to her husband's impotence. The meaning of "protecting the marriage" was not based in a belief in any theoretical orientation—in this case, Milan family therapy—or viewed as representing an ultimate truth or a better way of understanding the depression. Rather, the ascribed meaning emerged from the collaborative process of the interview, validated the client's experience, and fit or matched the content of the client's presentation. Although the therapist did not believe in the invariant truth of a Milan view *across* cases, the therapist did believe that a Milan view offered a credible and *plausible* explanation in this particular case.

In addition to the true versus different meanings distinction, interpretation and therapist-ascribed meaning are different in terms of goals (Duncan & Solovey, 1989). The immediate objective of interpretation is to promote insight or increase client understanding and self-awareness. Interpretation is useful because it leads to insight, and insight is seen as a key for better psychological living and a precursor for effective behavior change (Johnson, 1981). The immediate, or short-term, goal is insight, and it is then expected that behavior change will ultimately occur.

While the ultimate, or long-range, goal may be behavior change, the pursuit of understanding is sometimes a long-term process and an end in and of itself. Therapist-ascribed meaning, conversely, is primarily and specifically designed to create a context for an immediate meaning revision or behavior change in relation to the presenting problem. Therapist-ascribed meaning, therefore, is different from interpretation in that the immediate goal of the former is problem experience revision, as opposed to the long-term, or ultimate, goal of interpretation. If the problematic experience persists despite the different meaning ascribed by the therapist, that particular meaning is not considered useful, and another one may be offered. It is the behavioral outcome that determines the utility of an ascribed meaning rather than the client's verbal acceptance; increased awareness is only helpful if it leads to a change in the presenting problem.

If Sandra's depression would have persisted without change, the therapist-ascribed meaning would not have been viewed as useful by the therapist—even given Sandra's initial positive reception. Similarly, the connection between the depression and her husband's impotence would have been seen as helpful only if the client was enabled to *do* something about her situation or *feel* noticeably less depressed and acknowledge it. The therapist is always ready to allow ascribed meanings to fade away if they are not helpful, regardless of how they may initially seem to fit. Such was not the case with Sandra. Sandra returned to session two and announced that she was telling her husband that she was leaving and that she was prepared to end the marriage. She added that her depression was nonexistent when she wasn't thinking about her husband and their lack of sexual intimacy. Sandra decided that it was high time for action. Sandra and Gene returned in session three and began working on the impotence problem.

Therapist-Ascribed Meaning: Selection of Content

One of the advantages of a process, rather than a content, view of psychotherapy is the flexibility it allows the therapist. As the client describes the presenting problem, and therapeutic conversation unfolds and expands that description, a meaning system surrounding the complaint emerges. This emergent reality or meaning system provides the raw material for the therapist selection of content that may permit the client to reorganize perception and experience. The formal content selected by the therapist is dependent upon the idiosyncratic content focus of the client, as well as the specific clinical situation and its historical presentation.

The particular formal content chosen and the meaning formulated from it is a collaborative choice, given that it involves both the client's and therapist's input into the process. The conversation may lead to the client's making a distinction or connection, which evolves to the point where the therapist may punctuate that process with a therapist-ascribed meaning. It is not the correct or even corrective nature of formal content that is important, but rather the relationship between the formal content and the client's presentation that gives formal content its therapeutic potential.

The therapeutic relationship provides a safe place for clients to experiment with alternative meanings and risk revisions of those meanings and experiences that they find problematic. The therapist needs to be cautious about the formal content selected and be aware of the reality that he or she is constructing with the client. Formal content should expand the client's frame of reference and have the potential to include different options for the client or less distressing meaning attached to the problem.

Formal content, as a general rule, that pathologizes the problem or defines the problem as having restricted options should be avoided. In other words, the therapist should not introduce formal content unless that content provides a therapist-recognized opportunity for client change. Formal content may be selected from four sources to enable a therapist-ascribed meaning that validates client experience and offers a different perspective of the problem: (1) generic response patterns (2) specific clinical areas (3) specific theoretical orientation and (4) content *solely* arising from the client.

Generic Response Patterns

Generic response patterns describe culturally typical patterns or phases of response to developmental transitions or incidental crises that may have an organizing quality for the client. Generic response patterns can be used to expand the context in which the client experiences the problem, thereby providing the opportunity for the revision of meaning. In the following case, the client's presentation suggested that formal content from grief work be used to help a grieving mother reorganize her ongoing struggle with her son's death.

Evelyn, the branch manager of a loan company, was referred by her supervisor because of complaints by fellow employees about her moodiness, irritability, and intimidating style of management. Evelyn had been suspended and was being considered for termination.

During the initial interview, Evelyn stated that she was a competitive, hard-driving manager and that her branch had won all the sales competitions in the past 2 years. Evelyn stated also that she certainly had no intention of abusing her employees and wanted to correct any problems of which she was unaware. Evelyn discussed her work situation and the inherent stressors and contradictions from upper management that she had to endure on a daily basis. She also said that she was feeling like things were getting out of control in her life, as they did when her infant son died 3 years previously. When asked if she thought there was a connection between the death of her son and the moodiness, Evelyn replied that she wondered about that herself on many occasions

Evelyn told the story about how her son had been born with a serious cardiac defect and had had a shunt implanted, and about how 4 days before his scheduled surgery, the shunt had clotted and Brad had died in her arms. Evelyn said she took the death hard and was still struggling with it. She also said that she and her husband looked at other 3-year-old boys of friends and neighbors and tried to imagine how Brad would have looked, what he would have said and done. Evelyn was very angry with herself for giving Brad defective genes, at the doctors for not scheduling the operation sooner, and that her dreams for her son had died.

The therapist asked if Evelyn and her husband had ever talked to anyone about the process and work of grieving, and she said that they had not. They did attend a group for grieving parents briefly but found it too depressing. The therapist briefly explained some concepts about the process of grieving and the work of grieving, especially as it pertained to the emancipation from the deceased person. The therapist suggested that Evelyn's moodiness and problem at work could be an expression of her anger and other feelings about Brad's death.

Evelyn returned 2 weeks later and related how their 6-year-old son, Brett, was with her when they inadvertently drove by the cemetery where Brad was buried. Brett began asking questions about dying, the cause of Brad's death, what it meant to be buried, etc. Evelyn said this really took her and her husband by surprise and, in a very touching way, told the therapist how they tried to answer Brett's questions the best they could. They also visited the grave with flowers they had all gathered. Evelyn said that explaining Brad's death and attempting to make it concrete for Brett had helped her and her husband let go of Brad, and their dreams for him, a little bit more. She said that for the first time, they really had dealt with their son's death as a family. Evelyn returned for three more sessions and specifically addressed her interpersonal style with fellow employees. Her employer noted a significant decrease in her moodiness, which Evelyn attributed to the grieving of Brad's death.

The therapist saw Evelyn's connection between what was currently happening and her experience when she lost her son, Brad, as an opportunity to introduce the content of "grief." The grieving process provided an organizing framework for her to address the work problem. Based upon Evelyn's presentation of formal content and the connection of her son's death with her job predicament, the therapist ascribed the meaning of the emancipation process to Evelyn's moodiness and problems at work, which enabled the work problems to improve as she worked through the emancipation process. The meaning of grief validated the client's experience of her moodiness in a nonblaming way that permitted her to risk dealing with both her son's death and the problems at work.

Specific Clinical Areas

Sometimes clients present with discrete, clearly delineated concerns. With some complaints, the efficacy of a particular approach, specific conceptualization, or technique is well documented and may provide useful ways of organizing the client's problem. Content from a specific clinical source may be utilized as a primary framework if the client's description of the problem matches a particular content area. A therapist's use of specific clinical content may facilitate exploration of the problem and expand its context to include revisions of meaning helpful for problem resolution.

Pam, a 32-year-old mother of two, was seen in an emergency room for an attack of reflux esophagitis. She thought she was dying of a heart attack and panicked. Her subsequent experiences with anxiety and panic led to her being medicated for anxiety and depression by her family physician. Still experiencing anxiety, Pam monitored her body, and every ache and pain frightened her, precipitating more anxiety and panic. Headaches meant possible brain tumors, a tender underarm meant possible breast cancer, a sore shin meant bone cancer. Her physician checked out each complaint and tried to reassure her that she was fine. Although she knew physically she was not seriously ill, she continued to experience anxiety and still felt something was terribly wrong with her. Her physician recommended therapy.

Validating the reasonableness of these fears, given the scare Pam experienced with the esophagitis attack, the therapist offered the explanation that anxiety was a biologically necessary reaction. He then asked if she would like to know more about the physiology of anxiety so that she could better determine for herself what she was somatically experiencing. Pam replied that she would. The therapist explained the biological/chemical nature of anxiety, describing the structure of the autonomic nervous system and the arousal process. The therapist also discussed the causes of cardiovascular diseases and myocardial infarction symptoms to differentiate them from the reflux esophagitis and the anxiety/panic she experienced (Wilson, 1986).

Pam also wanted to discuss the medications (Prozac and Xanax) she had been prescribed. The therapist explained the basic differences between antidepressant and anxiolytic medications. Pam stated that she was only depressed as a result of the esophagitis and the resulting anxiety. By the second session, she had discontinued Prozac, after consulting with her physician. Also, Pam read a book about anxiety and watched a video tape that suggested behavioral ways of controlling anxiety. Although still using Xanax, she wanted to explore nonmedical means of controlling her anxiety. She had already begun listening to a relaxation cassette tape. The therapist and Pam then collaboratively built a program of "overcoming anxiety by choice" (Emery & Campbell, 1986) that included accepting her anxiety (as anxiety), watching her anxiety, and acting as if she was not anxious.

In the third session, Pam provided an example of how she calmed herself one night when her husband was away on a business trip without using medication. She experimented in calming herself a few times, and, over time, Pam gained confidence in learning to control her anxiety/

panic without medication. Although she did experience minor reoccur-rences of reflux esophagitis (controlled mainly by diet), her anxiety was no longer distressful.

Pam's reaction to the reflux esophagitis and her "feeling that something is terribly wrong with me" matched the specific clinical content area of anxiety/panic disorders. The therapist validated this experience as a scare that would result in anxiety/panic, ascribed the meaning of anxiety as a biologically necessary reaction to fear, and utilized the client's avid interest in acquiring knowledge about anxiety/panic experiences as a possible way for her to put her somatic complaints in perspective. Validated in her experience, Pam accepted this revision of meaning based in anxiety/panic disorder and expanded the context of her experience by reading and watching a video tape on the subject. This allowed her to step away from this very frightening experience and learn to cope with both her physical condition and her anxiousness without medication.

Specific Theoretical Orientations

Because no particular theoretical orientation must be used exclusively, meaning may be ascribed from any content area, as long as it is consistent with the client's constructed reality as it emerges in the therapeutic conversation. Several specific theoretical orientations were selected for use in the following case.

Ted

Ted, a 41-year-old executive, presented with complaints of anxiety and periodic panic attacks. Explaining his problem in detail, he was unable to identify any precipitating event or speculate upon any cause for the anxiety; in fact, he reported that everything in his life was going well. He clearly stated that his goal was to identify options that might permit understanding and control of his anxiety. He would then evaluate their merits and choose an action plan to implement. The client was somewhat familiar with different treatment modalities as a result of a class he had taken. Ted's desire to understand his anxiety and his familiarity with treatment options were respected and were instrumental in the therapist's selection of content.

The therapist told Ted that there were many options to consider and that he needed Ted's help. Ted replied by asking what the options were, to which the therapist responded:

"None of these options I'm about to offer is the truth, with a capital 'T,' but are, rather, a few of the many different ways that the various schools of therapy might suggest. A psychoanalytic therapist might suggest that your anxiety problem is a surface manifestation of an underlying, unresolved conflict, and represents a defense against this conflict coming to your conscious mind. Hence, he or she would believe that the unresolved conflict could probably be best understood by the exploration of your childhood and your relationship with your parents.

A behavioral therapist might suggest that your anxiety is a learned physiological response to certain situational events that is somehow being reinforced or rewarded in the environment. A behavioral therapist would advocate the learning of a relaxation technique so that you can have a coping response to respond to those situations instead of your current response of anxiety and panic attacks.

An existential therapist might suggest that your anxiety represents a message to you that you have lost meaning, or a sense of purpose in your life—that things that contained meaning for you no longer serve as motivating factors or a source of fulfillment. This existential dilemma is basically a struggle that we all must face—attempting to find meaning in a world with no apparent meaning. The treatment would consist of an exploration of your inner self and the consideration of the issues of freedom, responsibility, and your authorship of your own destiny.

A family therapist might say that your anxiety is, in some way, protective to your marriage and is a nonverbal message of some sort that you are attempting to convey to your wife about some aspect of your relationship. In other words, it may be stabilizing your marriage and defining or redefining the basic nature of your relationship. A family therapist might suggest that your anxiety may be best addressed through marital therapy."

Ted replied by asking how he would know which option was best. The therapist then asked Ted to spend 15–30 minutes making himself feel as anxious as he could to see if any of the options made sense in the context of the actual anxiety experience.

In the next session, Ted reported that he had attempted the exercise and was unable to make himself very anxious, his anxiety had diminished, and he had experienced no panic attacks. He added that he had figured out what the anxiety was about, which permitted him to take different action. After much consideration during his attempts to follow the prescription, subsequently he concluded that the anxiety was related to the boredom of his job and the lack of romance in his marriage. The client then contacted an employment recruiter, as well as discussed the lack of romance in his marriage with his wife, who was relieved to finally address a heretofore unspoken issue.

Formal content was selected both from a specific clinical content area and several specific orientations, given Ted's presentation of his anxiety problem. The clinical content area of "anxiety" was the obvious choice, given Ted's presenting complaints. This content area provided a conceptual framework that was consistent with Ted's view of the problem situation. Recall Ted's initial expressed desire to explore several possible causes and solutions to his complaint. In service of that desire, the therapist presented psychoanalytic, behavioral, existential, and family therapy explanations for the anxiety.

Client response to a particular content area indicates the fit, or lack thereof, with the client's meaning system. To the extent to which fit occurs, it directs the pursuit of any given content area in the therapeutic conversation. The overriding goal is to alter the meaning or context of the problem process in the direction of improvement. Content matches client circumstances, rather than tailoring client circumstances to the therapist's orientation.

After Ted reported the change in his anxiety, as well as the steps he had taken to help himself in his job and marriage, the therapist facilitated a discussion of the client's newly acquired meaning by asking questions encouraging the detailed articulation of how and why the change came about. Ted reported that, for too long, he had resigned himself to the fact that his life was dull and somewhat pointless. He also commented that he had accepted that his relationship with his wife was little more than a functional arrangement. Encouraged by his wife's response and his own initiative regarding his job, Ted concluded by asserting that he felt relieved to be back in control and pleased that he was able to overcome his resignation to an unfulfilling life.

Ted believed there was no reason for the anxiety and tried to discount it, or will it away. The client's meaning system of restricted possible solutions and invalidation was challenged by a smorgasbord of possible explanations. The combination of a competing experience (suggesting that he purposefully experience anxiety) and many possible alternate ascriptions of meaning allowed the *client* to interpret the anxiety in a way that was most helpful to him. The therapist simply wanted to "menu" many ascriptions of alternate meaning for the anxiety and to let Ted pick his own ascription. This set a context for change by having Ted search for his own meaning and solution, which he ultimately did.

The meanings ascribed by the therapist flowed from the direct request by the client and were delivered in such a way to encourage Ted to challenge the invalidation of his "no reason" meaning system. The meanings were not imposed by the therapist, but rather chosen by the client—an empowering experience, given that the client creatively and idiosyncratically combined the existential and family therapy content areas in a way that enabled Ted to make changes in his marriage and work.

Peg, Dan, and Sam

An intact family of three sought therapy for "school phobia." Sam, the 10-year-old son, had not attended school more than once weekly in the prior month. With a hint of anger in her voice, Mother (Peg) reported that each day she arose before the others, completed leftover chores, prepared the family's breakfast, and prepared Sam for school. Mother then departed for work, leaving Sam alone to wait a half hour for the bus. Within the half hour, Sam would phone mother at work, complaining of nausea. Mother would return home to minister to Sam, who, on occasion, would vomit.

Peg's resentment ultimately played a big role in the selection of content. The content and language of a particular approach (Madanes, 1981) was utilized because of the therapist's perception of Mother's anger and the inequality of responsibility that seemed apparent. The selection of this content was predicated by the client presentation, rather than the belief in the inherent truth of the Madanes model. (The Madanes model discusses child problems as metaphorical expressions of parental difficulties and unresolved conflicts.)

T: There are certainly a lot of ways to look at a problem like this. Some therapists might say, and this may sound a bit crazy so please bear with me, that Sam's school phobia problem, his getting sick to his stomach in the morning, is a metaphorical expression of unexpressed anger between his parents.

P: What do you mean? [Looking interested.]

T: Well, again, this is just one way of looking at this problem—that Sam gets sick in the morning, preventing him from going to school, is a metaphorical expression of Mom being sick and tired of carrying the whole load. After all, both of your jobs are equally important, yet it is always Mom who must interrupt her work routine and come home, while Dad is able to work and not be bothered. Not to mention that it is Mom who must also be responsible for keeping the house, fixing the meals, etc. In essence, then, and this may seem far-fetched, when Sam throws up, he's doing it more for Mom than for himself.

P: That's great! [Laughing for a while.] You know, I haven't told Dan about my resentment for all this.

D: What should we do?

T: To let Sam see that he is no longer needed to express Mom's unexpressed resentment, it may be helpful for you, Dan, to help a bit more around the house—but, more importantly, it may more strongly convey the message to Sam if you are the one that he calls in the morning when he is sick. Are you willing to try that?

D: Of course, anything that will help.

T: It also may help, Peg, if you monitor your anger and let Dan know when your load gets too heavy.

P: That sounds like a good idea.

It was the mother's affect or emotional experience surrounding the presenting problem (i.e., anger) as well as the specific circumstances of the occurrence of the problem (i.e., inequitable home and parental responsibilities) that became salient in the selection of the ascribed meaning. The different meaning was selected, not because the therapist believed it to be a necessarily true or a better meaning, but rather as constituting an attempt to offer different information to encourage the client construction of a more helpful meaning system, that is, one in which problem improvement could occur. Likewise, the Madanes conceptualization was selected because it seemed to fit the presentation of the family and their feedback in response to it. After delivering the suggestion that Sam call Dad instead of Mom, Sam replied, "I guess I won't be staying home any more." At follow-up, this indeed, was the case.

Content Solely Generated by the Client

Many revisions of meaning incorporate content produced solely by the client. Most discussions of reframing use examples that are based in the client's presented content. Validating the client's experience, using questions to expand the context of the client's experience, and getting an interactional description of what others are saying and doing are essential to the ascription of alternate meaning. The search is for meaning that holds a different connotation than originally ascribed by the client, which therefore leads to different remedial action. The meaning expressed by the client is neither discounted nor confronted, but rather validated and then expanded or altered to include the possibility of a more helpful connotation.

The following case exemplifies this process. The informal content presented by the client was all that was utilized; no other formal content from any other source was added. By using a simple ascription, the context was expanded to include a different meaning, which the client chose to accept.

Joan sought therapy after being advised by her physician to stop drinking. She was concerned that she did not have the will power to quit drinking, because of her experiences growing up in her family of origin. Joan was extremely angry and bitter toward her mother, who had abused her both emotionally and physically. Joan reported that her mother was an alcoholic who had married seven times. With much anger and disgust in her voice, Joan stated that the reason she felt she could not stop drinking was that her mother had damaged her emotionally.

The theme of Joan's anger and the cause-and-effect relationship between her mother's abuse and her drinking repeatedly surfaced in the interview. Joan reported several previous therapy attempts at resolving her anger/hate toward her mother; she seemed, at times, to be almost proud that each therapy attempt had failed, leaving her just as hateful as before.

Given the intensity of the presentation of Joan's anger, as well as her strongly held belief that she was destined to drink because of her mother, the therapist chose to utilize her anger and belief as ingredients in the intervention. To counter and interrupt Joan's use of her anger and resentment in self-destructive ways, the therapist ascribed a different meaning to Joan's alcohol abuse, to help her use her bitterness and anger as a source of strength to stop drinking. It was hoped that the different meaning would serve as an expanded context for different actions regarding her drinking.

The therapist said:

"A lot of people who are children of alcoholics show them respect by developing a similar or worse problem. It may be that by developing your problem, unconsciously you let your mother know that she has nothing to worry about—you'll never show her up by rising above her. Imitation is the greatest form of respect—your mother was alcoholic, so, out of respect, you have developed a drinking problem. What do you suppose your mother would do if you suddenly lost your drinking problem and demonstrated that you were capable of doing something constructive for yourself? It may be that at some level she would resent you for showing her that you no longer fit into the family mold. It may be that you recognize this at some level and such a recognition may form the unconscious basis for your continued drinking."

The therapist ended the session by telling the client to call if she wanted to pursue the discussion further. She called 3 months later and reported that she had stopped drinking after the session and had been sober ever since. She was now concerned about a marital problem and was seeking consultation for it. The therapist worked with Joan for two additional sessions, and her marital problem improved. At termination, Joan reported that her relationship with her mother was better since Joan had stopped drinking and that she had made other productive changes in her life.

The therapist-ascribed meaning of "showing respect" was not viewed as representing an ultimate truth or better way of understanding her drinking problem. Rather, the therapist designed the ascribed meaning based on the client's presentation in the hopes of influencing the client to take immediate and different action about her drinking. The case of Joan was not taken lightly; the meaning was ascribed after a thorough research of her perceptions of previous experiences in therapy and her meaning system related to her mother. This case represents an order of intervention that falls on the negative side of our responses to clients. It was Joan's seemingly unshakeable belief that her mother was selfish and our respect for previous failed attempts to develop a better relationship between her and her mother that led the therapist to try something different. Furthermore, the intervention, however it may appear, recognized and validated how Joan perceived her mother's negative treatment of her. Any attempt to present her mother in a more benign way may have trivialized her experience of her mother. The intervention seemed to provide input that helped Joan organize her negative experience of her mother in a positive way to stop drinking. The intervention not only respected Joan's meaning system, but also cooperated with her reason for entering therapy. "Showing respect" validated her meaning system regarding her alcoholic mother, and offered a different perspective that allowed Joan to do the work necessary to stop drinking.

Therapist Role in the Ascription of Alternative Meaning

Although therapist style is idiosyncratically determined and interpreted within the context of the therapeutic relationship, therapists' understanding of their role makes the difference between the "technique" of reframing and the collaborative revision of meaning.

Previous discussions in Chapter 5 regarding delivery are also applicable to revision of meaning interventions. That discussion emphasized the therapeutic relationship as cooperative and collaborative, and as *the* vehicle for any intervention to occur. In ascribing different meanings, we do not *pretend* to believe the alternative meanings; we take very seriously the task of trying to find something in the client's meaning system that we can genuinely relate to, and then build on that bridge to select and deliver a revised meaning. We are opportunists who not only look for seeds within the client's realm of experience that can be nurtured to revise the meaning of that experience, but we also seek respectful ways to do this.

Clients have multiple pathways to meaning revision and it is unknown how people will respond to a given revision of meaning. When a client does not accept the revision or it is not helpful, it is not interpreted as "pathological" in terms of "denial" or "resistance." We deny "denial" and resist "resistance" as concepts that preclude effective delivery of revised meaning. Searching for other opportunities for revision of meaning and other opportunities for the respectful offering of that meaning continues as long as the client is willing to engage in the process and the therapist remains flexible.

When we say "offer" revisions of meaning, we mean the tentative and qualified suggestion of an alternate meaning. The spirit of beneficent experimentation also applies to therapist-ascribed meaning. In delivering in-session revisions of meaning, it is simply suggested that the person consider the revision of meaning. A revision of meaning must never be given with an "I have a solution to your problem" frame. We are not prescribing specific meanings to be taken as literal truth, but rather are suggesting alternatives to expand the context of the experiences clients share with us.

SUMMARY

This chapter has presented the revision of meaning strategies of empowering client-ascribed meaning and therapist-ascribed meaning. These meaning-oriented interventions were described as representing a process of the ebb and flow of ideas occurring in the context of the therapeutic dialogue that ultimately culminates in the ascription of a revised meaning by the client or therapist. Client-ascribed meaning was distinguished from insight in that (1) insight is therapist generated and emanates from a particular theoretical frame of reference, whereas client-ascribed meaning is client-generated; and (2) insight is a precondition of change, whereas client-ascribed meaning occurs during change or afterwards. Therapist-ascribed meaning was compared to reframing and differentiated from it by (1) therapist-ascribed meaning represents the culmination or punctuation of a collaborative process between the client and therapist; (2) therapist-ascribed meaning is an explicit therapist behavior that both validates the client's experience *and* offers an alternative perspective; and (3) therapist-ascribed meaning utilizes frames or meanings from any possible source, including other therapy approaches. Finally, therapist-ascribed meaning and interpretation were contrasted by (1) therapist-ascribed meaning is intended to present different ways of viewing client concerns, whereas interpretation seeks to present a particular and perhaps inherently better way based on the therapist's orientation; and (2) therapist-ascribed meaning seeks to promote an immediate problem experience revision, whereas interpretation is intended to promote insight and ultimately a change in the presenting problem.

7   Case Study: "The Loser"

NOW that the reader has experience with the empirical influences, theoretical foundations, pragmatic assumptions, and clinical application of the proposed approach, this chapter presents excerpts from each session of a case that hopefully integrates the different aspects into a coherent whole. Actual session dialogue is presented and accompanied by commentary that explains the therapist's actions.

The case study allows the reader to track with the therapeutic process in much the same fashion that observing a case behind a one-way mirror permits. The therapist–client conversation provides the "live" information. The accompanying commentary represents the discussion and case planning behind the mirror.

Hal was referred by his company's employee assistance program (EAP). The only information the therapist had before the interview was that Hal had a "near" suicide attempt, experienced occasional suicidal ideation, and was depressed.

SESSION ONE

Excerpt One

T: What brings you here to see me today?

C: I've got so much to tell. About a year ago we discovered my son had dyslexia and it was a long, drawn-out process just to get the testing done.

T: Yes.

C: And when we were going through the discovery process—finding out what could be done, going out and getting books and everything, there was a little pamphlet put out by the—I think it was—the National Education, U.S. Government, and I read the pamphlet, and I felt like I was reading a case history on myself. So I had the testing done and found out that I have learning disabilities too. And I was sitting there talking with the tester—we were going through everything—and she suggested that I get counseling—talk to somebody—because of the frustration, depression, anxieties I've gone through. I never told them about it, but it came out in the test. So I went to the EAP counselor and she referred me here.

T: O.K. So, can you describe for me some of the frustrations and anxieties you experience as the result of that.

C: The frustration was constantly failing. Anything I do, I fail. Like I told the EAP counselor, I've got it down to a science. Anywhere I go, anything I do, it blows up in my face. It gets bad sometimes, real bad—and it's getting more and more and more. It keeps building up.

T: This is kind of a dumb question, but how do you know that you're depressed?

C: I don't look at anything positive—I always look at the negative side.

T: You have a pessimistic outlook?

C: Very. I used to have an optimistic outlook.

T: How long ago did you have an optimistic outlook?

C: Oh, that was a long, long time ago—it must have been 8 years ago.

T: O.K. So you've been depressed for 8 years?

C: At least.

T: So you've had a pessimistic outlook for 8 years.

C: Progressively. It wasn't one day I was optimistic, and the next day I was pessimistic—things just progressed until now. Nothing looks good to me any more. I don't know if the EAP counselor told you, I've had suicidal thoughts.

T: Any recently?

C: The last one wasn't too long ago. I was sitting in the bathroom, and I had a bottle of pills in my hand—out of the bottle. There was a good 10 to 15 of them there. But I stopped—I stopped myself.

T: How were you able to do that?

C: I keep thinking of my son, what he'd go through, what teasing and hard times he'd go through when everybody found out his old man committed suicide. I keep thinking about that, but one day I might not think about it and just go ahead and do it.

T: Things must have really gotten bad for you.

Commentary

Hal begins to tell his story, and the therapist pursues the nature of the problem, looking for an interactional description, meaning revision opportunities, and openings for validation of Hal's experience. The sequence rapidly progresses to Hal's recent suicide attempt. The near attempt presented the therapist the opportunity to highlight how Hal was able to stop himself, as well as validate how distressing Hal's life had become for him to consider suicide. Hal continues to unfold his story and the mutual exchange of meaning between Hal and the therapist creates a context for further validation and the attainment of more information.

Excerpt Two

C: I never did like this area.

T: It's kind of hard to like. No one comes here for vacation.

C: I'm glad somebody agrees. I like wide open spaces—I like the West.

T: When did you come back?

C: About 3 years last December. We moved from New Mexico to Florida so I could work with some horses—thoroughbreds—but that was seasonal work, and I got fired 2 months after we went there. Then my dad offered to move us here, and so we came back, and he bought us a trailer and has done everything for us . . . I'm 31 years old, and I'm living off my dad. That's what bugs me a lot. I should be making a living for myself and for my family, and I'm not doing it.

T: So your ability as a breadwinner is not very good, in your estimation, because your dad essentially supported you.

C: Right. He's supporting us now.

T: How so now?

C: Working at a loan company, you don't make very much.

T: So he's subsidizing you now on a monthly basis.

C: Yes. Probably around $300 a month.

T: Nice dad, but you probably feel bad with every dollar.

C: I feel pretty bad. I have to go and get the checks from him—it's kind of degrading.

T: Yes. And he doesn't ask for anything in return?

C: He tries to run our life a little bit.

T: O.K., so there are some strings attached.

C: But half the time I don't even listen to him.

T: So you feel that you have some autonomy.

C: I have to feel that way. If I felt obligated to take his advice and use it the way he says to use it, I probably wouldn't even be here. I probably would have been long gone. Either I would have committed suicide, or I would have run away. Just plain out and out run away. I wouldn't care who followed me or who came with me.

T: What ever possessed you to come back?

C: I got fired from a job out there for letting a $75 check pay. It was marked "stop payment," and I was used as a scapegoat.

T: You were working in a bank?

C: Um huh. And the only job I could get after that was working for a pizza place as a driver, and I didn't feel like there was a future for me anywhere in Santa Fe, and we decided to move to Florida to work with horses. I was a hot walker down there, I was about ready to become a groomer, and they moved all the horses to another ranch, and I was left out in the cold. I wasn't even given the choice of whether I wanted to go or not. I was just gone. And then we came back here when there wasn't any jobs that I could find in Florida.

T: So you found one at the loan company. Do you like it there?

C: The money situation just doesn't work.

T: So you've been looking for other work?

C: Um huh. I have my application in as an accounting clerk. I'm just waiting for some calls now.

T: That gives you a shot at a lot better-paying job.

C: I think it starts out at about $16,000 a year.

T: Do you think that would be the cure of your ills?

C: Some of it. If I could start making a somewhat better living, bringing in more money, I think that would help me a lot. But you know, the other aspect, I need a skill or an education too to be able to bring in more money. And that's what's been bothering me all along. I consider myself to be of average intelligence, if not above average, but when it comes to school or taking a test—forget it. I can sit down and talk with somebody until we're blue in the face and put up a good argument, even though I never cracked a book on the subject, but if you sit down and ask me to take a test on that same argument, I couldn't put it down on paper for you. It's like there's a block between my mind and my hand. I couldn't even think it out for you. Essay tests are forget it.

T: And mainly it's because of your learning disability.

C: That's what's coming out now. I was so relieved when I found that out. I was *so* relieved; I thought there was something drastically wrong.

T: That you were stupid or something?

C: Yes. Or retarded or something. It was like there was somebody inside me trying to get out, but couldn't find the door. You have 10,000 doors on each wall, and you have four walls. That's the way I feel half the time, and I can't get anybody else to realize that.

T: What have you tried so far to get over the depression or pessimistic outlook?

C: Ignore it. That doesn't work.

T: Not too well. That's kind of a John Wayne strategy.

C: Let's see. I've tried to ignore it; I've tried to work myself into a happier mood. Sometimes I sit there at my machine and sing, and everybody puts their headphones on or starts howling. That's it.

T: What does your wife suggest for you to do?

C: She has no suggestions. She doesn't know what to do for me.

T: She's frustrated with you.

C: I think she's frustrated with my moods, yes. My mood swings. One day I'll be a happy-go-lucky guy and you can have fun with me, and the next day I'll be so far down you have to look under the rug to find me.

T: What's your dad suggested that you do?

C: He doesn't know.

T: He doesn't know you're depressed?

C: He knows I'm depressed. He's suggested I go out and look for other jobs. I had an application in at the post office to take the test, and that came up the same day as my final interview with the tester, and it was either/or, not both. He wanted me to go take the test and reschedule the interview. I thought the interview was more important—that's one of the times I didn't listen to him, and he went into a tirade on that one. He thought I should have been at the post office taking the test.

T: So his view is that if you'd get out there and hump and find a better job, you'd be all right.

C: Um huh.

T: Has he given you any other advice about your pessimism or depression or ways to make yourself feel better, that kind of stuff?

C: No. He listens to me. We talk out things a lot of times, but he feels that if I could get out there and hump, find a better job, then all our worries would be over.

T: O.K. When the going gets tough, the tough get going—that kind of thing?

C: Um huh. He's very much into competition. He was an accountant at the base and retired a lieutenant colonel.

T: Do you salute him? [said humorously]

C: Sometimes I feel like it. Especially when he gets in some of those moods, yes. At times he orders people around. I let it go in one ear and out the other.

T: You don't let it bother you that much. Has anybody else given you any suggestions or advice about things to try to make you feel better? What did the EAP counselor say?

C: She just suggested I try more in-depth counseling—that I should come here because she really didn't feel like she could help me in the three to five sessions they could offer.

T: She didn't make any other suggestions?

C: Not that I can remember.

T: So your wife has not really made any suggestions.

C: No.

T: Your dad wants you to go out and get a better job.

C: Um huh.

T: And you have tried to ignore it and sometimes tried to "sing" your way through it, so to speak. Have any of these things worked?

C: No.

T: What's your mother suggested that you do?

C: My mother's a very religious person. She wants me to go to church, and I've tried that trip before and it doesn't work. I've always felt like I was on the outside looking in, everywhere I go, every organization I've ever been in. I'm the person in the group that everybody finds easy to ignore. And you find one of those in every group anywhere.

T: And it's always you.

C: It's always—I'm one of the ones. I'm a loser.

T: You're a loser.

C: That's the way I feel. That's basically the way I feel. I really feel like a loser. In high school I was a loser and a loner—I had one friend in the 3 years I was here in high school. He moved when his dad retired. Since then I've had one other good friend. I'm a loner, by myself most of the time. My parents thought I was real lazy.

T: Can't get Hal to do anything, can't get him to work in school. And that's the way you grew up.

C: That's the way I grew up. Until I finally became lazy. Just like one day, you think I'm lazy, O.K., I'll be lazy. That's the way I grew up. I had a hard time learning to read—they thought I just wasn't working, wasn't trying hard enough.

T: If you'd only put your mind to it, you'd be able to do it, right?

C: Um huh. Very familiar statements. If you would concentrate on it, you could do it. And I'd be sitting there concentrating on it for 3 hours, and I still couldn't do it. But they didn't see that.

T: A rotten way to grow up.

C: Um huh.

T: Your son isn't going to grow up that way.

C: No, he's never going to be that way. I will never do that to him. Because I can see in him what I went through. I can see where his mind's at, what he's trying to do, and he tries, I can see that he really tries. But at times he just can't get it, and I know how that feeling is. But now he's trying, and now he's getting it. And that feeling of success is a rush, especially where he's at—I know where he's at. When you succeed in one thing, it's party time. That's the way I feel. It comes few and far between.

T: For you now especially?

C: Um huh.

T: Do you have a pessimistic or negative outlook every day, all day? You mentioned that sometimes you're happy-go-lucky.

C: Not every day. Maybe 2, 3 days out of the week.

T: You're happy-go-lucky or pessimistic?

C: Happy-go-lucky. And it's usually the weekend, Friday, Saturday, and Sunday.

T: Fancy that! You're not at work, you're at home with your family.

C: I feel pretty good about myself on the weekends.

T: What would be an indication to you that things were beginning to move in the right direction, as far as your depression? What would be a sign to you that you were initiating the right step in the right direction? Not all the way there, or even a part of the way there, but beginning to get there. How would you know that?

C: I don't know. It's been with me for so long that I don't know. Eight years is a long time.

T: Yes it is. It's a long, long time.

C: I don't know where it would begin. It's just one of those things. When the feeling starts happening right, when I see things go right, like when I put my hands into something, I can't even tell you.

T: All right. Would you be willing to give that some serious thought?

C: Sure.

Commentary

Hal shares his story of repeated failures and invalidation experiences growing up, which led him to the conclusion that he is a loser—probably the ultimate example of a person whose story is itself invalidating. The therapist began by pursuing an interactional description of Hal's depression. During that process, Hal revealed an informal theory regarding his depression that was historically based on his childhood academic experiences and others' view of him as lazy and incompetent. Hal's continued failure experiences only served to reinforce his view of himself as a loser.

Hal's feelings of depression and self-ascribed meaning of loser were embedded in a cycle of solution attempts characterized by ignoring his depression and trying to cheer himself up, only to be faced with the ongoing reality of working an unsatisfactory job and remaining financially dependent on his father. As the story unfolded, the therapist continued asking questions within the content limitations presented by Hal, and several themes emerged. Each of these themes was noted by the therapist as an opportunity that might lead to meaning revision. Hal seemed quite resentful of his father and felt degraded by his financial support and advice. Hal resented his father's advice even though he agreed that finding a different job might at least partially solve his problem.

Another theme that emerged was that Hal not only wanted a different job, but one in which he could experience job satisfaction as well. It seemed that Hal knew what he needed to do, but was stuck by his view of himself as loser, as well as by others' similar views. In many ways, Hal's meaning system regarding his situation and himself was already changing, given the recent information he received regarding the learning disability. This new information or variability may have set the stage for the evolution of a different meaning that did not include Hal's feelings of shame about his past failures. The theme of a different job combined with education provided perhaps another opportunity for the therapist to explore that could lead to the co-generation of new meanings and different remedial actions.

The exception to Hal's depression also revealed a path that could be followed. Hal identified that he was not depressed on the weekends, which not only brought to light that Hal was not depressed all the time, but also emphasized the depressing aspects of his job situation more emphatically.

The therapist's dilemma at this point was not a paucity of paths to follow, but rather which one of the many opportunities that were generated in the therapeutic conversation should be pursued further. The therapist wanted to interrupt Hal's solutions of ignoring his situation and trying to cheer himself up, as well as challenge his meaning system of himself as a loser. After consideration and a break to collect his thoughts, the therapist concluded that what seemed most important was to legitimize solidly Hal's feeling of depression and justify his view of himself as a loser, given Hal's life experience. Such a validation could enable Hal to expand his frame of reference to replace the invalidation of his own and others' description of him, and, perhaps, include proactive behaviors concerning his job and financial dependence on his father. Validation enhances common factors and sets the stage for rapid client change. If Hal remembers nothing else other than the therapist's message of outright justification of Hal's meaning system, then the first interview is a resounding success.

Excerpt Three

"First of all, given what you've told me so far, it's certainly not surprising to me that you're pessimistic. In fact, you're maybe more realistic than you are pessimistic. You had a few different jobs that have ended because of termination of the job, or they terminated you over something you did that they blamed you for and scapegoated you. You've tried some things, they've blown up in your face, you grew up your whole life with people telling you you're a lazy bum essentially. And you, knowing in one sense that's not true, but not being able to come to grips with that because you didn't have any framework to understand it till recently. You've had to move around to find work, then you come back here after having several failures, if you want to call them that, after a lifelong label of being lazy and incompetent and maybe a loser and you'll never go anywhere, or do anything, or be anybody. And you come here, which is proof positive, because then your old man takes you in. He buys you a trailer and he subsidizes your income, which is the same message—you're a loser, you'll never amount to anything, and I've still got to take care of you. I only know one way to respond to that, and that's by being depressed. You're working at a job that pays $11–12,000, and this day and time that's poverty. You're trying to raise a family on an impossible income. That's a big enough bummer in and of itself, I think. And to add on top of that you find out something very serious about your son. That he has a problem that has to be dealt with, and you went through that 6-month hassle on getting some resolution to that, which, I'm sure was, even at lowered expense, was not cheap, and now you have this eye doctor stuff going on and that continued pressure and expense. I guess all that's to say is that I'm not surprised at all that you are depressed. In fact, I would think you were a little bonzo if you weren't. A lot of people with the kind of life stressors you've had would be in the hospital or would have committed the act already. I think you are doing amazingly well, considering all the garbage you've had to deal with. And that's really undercutting the garbage of growing up and being told you're lazy and really having a learning disability and no one understanding that. It's no wonder you feel like a loser, because you were. You didn't get to experience things everybody else did, which were competence in reading and understanding. The things that sets off in a person is not good. And carrying that on as a lifestyle and then having things continually reinforce that, and failure at jobs, not really fitting in in organizations or clubs or work. So I think you'd be silly as hell to be optimistic, given your circumstance—Pollyannaish, I guess. I'd be concerned about you if you had an optimistic outlook now. I'd think you were nuts."

Commentary

The therapist validated Hal's experience, highlighted the impact of the events of Hal's life, and legitimized his feelings of depression. Throughout the validation, Hal responded with head nods and tearing eyes. Hal also responded with a very softly spoken, "Someone understands." In session two, the therapist checked out how things were going, was attentive to any indications of change, and pursued the themes described earlier in hopes of co-creating new meanings and evolving opportunities for heretofore unsaid descriptions, connections, implications, and distinctions.

SESSION TWO

Excerpt Four

T: Well, how's it been going?

C: Decently.

T: So does decently mean that it's different than it was before, or is it about the same?

C: It hasn't been any worse, let me put it that way. It seems to have leveled off a little bit.

T: Has anything happened to account for that?

C: Just getting things off my chest—being able to talk to somebody, that helps a lot.

T: When you say things are decent—they didn't get any worse—how did you know they didn't' get any worse, as far as the way you felt?

C: I didn't feel the safety valve close up on me—gum up on me—like before when I thought about doing it all, the safety valve felt gummed up. I couldn't release any of the pressure, the frustration. Now it seems like it's getting cleared—I can release some of the frustration just by simply talking and it's getting clearer and clearer.

Commentary

The therapist noticed a slight difference in Hal's affective presentation. Hal seemed more alive and less flat. The therapist pursued this perceived difference, being open to any serendipitous occurrences or possible client-ascribed meaning that could be unfolded and empowered. Hal labeled his current status as "decent" and attributed the "leveling off" to talking things out and releasing pressure and frustration. The validation may have paved the way for Hal to consider initiating some changes. The therapist followed Hal's lead, which moved the conversation toward the theme of Hal's job and Hal's recognized strength at machine repair. The ensuing conversation was not only significant because job satisfaction seemed like a relevant theme to explore regarding Hal's depression, but also because it represented the first self-validating aspect of Hal's story to this point in the therapy. The entire first session was characterized by Hal's failures and invalidations. Here he was in the second session discussing his successes and knowhow with machines.

Excerpt Five

C: I can do things other people can't, and it helps out the company at the same time too. A lot of the machines there are computerized, and I work on them so that we're not down as long or quite as often, even though I've never had the training in that field.

T: So you're pretty mechanically sharp?

C: With these particular machines, yes.

T: So they don't have to shut down and call a technician—they have you there.

C: Um huh.

T: I imagine your supervisor likes that when they don't go down.

C: She likes it quite a bit. She even writes it in my reviews, that I have above average knowledge of these machines. So when it does go down, they call me over, I look at it, and if I can't fix it, I'll write down what I think is wrong with the machine, and we staple it shut and call the technician. When he gets there, and we find out what's wrong, I open up my piece of paper to see if I was right or not. I'm ninety-five percent right.

T: Ninety-five percent? My gosh, that amazing.

C: I can just hear the machines. I hear them when things are going wrong, and I usually fix it before it goes wrong.

T: So you can do preventive kinds of things?

C: Um huh. I can hear when a belt—these little green belts like an O-ring—I can hear when it's stretching out. It starts squeaking a little bit. Nobody else hears the squeak. I call it Herman. Herman's coming back. And I'll shut down the machine, pull out my screwdrivers, and change the belt, and it's back to normal.

T: It sounds like there's one thing that people recognize your competence about in your life. If you look at all the different aspects of it, there's this area where other people see you have this skill or competence. You sound like a fireman—there's a problem, and I call you, and you come in and take care of it, which can be pretty satisfying stuff to do.

C: It's fun—I love it. I love it when I see things like that. It's like you see your accomplishment right then and there. It's not working on a project for a year and then you see your accomplishment, you see things going together right then.

T: When you see the machine come back on, you know you've done it.

C: And you know you've saved your company some money—you've saved your employer some money. Instead of the machine being down 2 hours, it's only down 2 minutes.

T: Had you ever been a technician or anything like that on any of your jobs?

C: No.

T: That's just been a natural affinity, not gotten through training.

C: Not working with the books. After 12 years of schooling and not being able to go anywhere, you kind of get scared of books. I've been thinking about training—going to school to get training—if I can find a tech school that has that special area where I can get some help, some tutoring.

T: That would help you get through because of your learning disability.

C: If I can find that special school, then I will. I'll go back to school for 2 years and get the training and go to work for a company, open up a little shop, work on something.

T: It would certainly be a lot more money.

C: It would be more satisfying. That's what I'm really looking for—something a little more satisfying.

T: Give you a sense of confidence.

C: When you can see your efforts coming together, you're making something work right. I talked to a couple schools since I was here last, and one of them was a fly-by-night. The office where they interviewed potential students seemed like a broom closet. Everything was in it. The other school cost $12,500 to go to school there for 2 years.

Commentary

Not only were things "decent" and had "leveled off," Hal also had investigated technical schools between sessions one and two. Hal's verbal report of a competence area (machine repair) combined with his actions to seek information about technical schools were not taken lightly by the therapist, but rather were viewed as indications that Hal was undergoing a meaning shift. Exploring the theme of job satisfaction and technical schools led to the reemergence of the topic of Hal's father and an unfolding of a relationship between Hal's loser ascriptions and his father's control over Hal's career choices.

Excerpt Six

C: My dad freaks out whenever I talk about doing anything other than regular college, even though I failed in college on two different tries.

T: You mean he tells you you shouldn't go to tech school?

C: Yes, he really looks down on any job that isn't white-collar professional. He's a real snob.

T: So he wouldn't approve of it if you went to tech school.

C: No way! One time I told him I was applying for a job in an automobile factory, and he told me if I did he was going to cut me off financially.

T: Pretty radical position.

C: He's good for threatening me with that if I do something he doesn't approve of. Another thing he's really bugging me about. He's looking at the learning disability as more of a block.

T: That it's a character problem?

C: Yes. Because every time he brings it up, it's more of a negative sense.

T: Like it's something you chose to do?

C: I don't know if it's that or if he's looking at it as a mental-retardation type thing.

T: Oh my gosh.

C: Something like that. I want to just grab him by the neck and slap his face.

T: Sure, that's quite a criticism.

C: He brings it up in a negative form, and he doesn't realize it's not. We found the cause of why I couldn't achieve in school and basically why I can't achieve in life, and now we can work on it, now we can go forward.

T: But he doesn't see it that way.

C: He sees it as a giant step backwards, falling down a cliff. And that's hard, trying to get him to understand it's not that at all. He is going to think of me as a loser unless I do things and succeed at what he thinks I should.

Commentary

Hal's father's strong negative stance toward tech school and Hal's learning disability seemed to be significant aspects of Hal's experience that perhaps were even obstacles to Hal's feeling better about himself or pursuing a career of his choice. Validating Hal's experience of himself as a loser and his feelings of depression seemed to help Hal begin to take some steps toward changing the dissatisfying aspects of his situation (e.g., investigate tech schools) as well as perhaps begin to view himself more benignly (e.g., strength at repair, 95% accuracy). The success of the validation, combined with the reemergent theme of Hal's resentment of his father's control, contributed to the therapist's decision to validate the difficulties Hal would face and had faced in any efforts to change his situation. The therapist chose to punctuate the emergent meaning regarding Hal's father and accomplish validation of Hal's difficulties in usurping his father's control by asking Hal to consider the disadvantages and obstacles he may face if he takes steps toward change.

The therapist pursued this path instead of suggesting a competing experience for two reasons. The first reason was that validation and the discussion of Hal's job dissatisfaction and his father seemed to result in client movement. Pursuing the disadvantages and obstacles to change would continue that process and perhaps would unfold new meanings leading to more change. The therapist was working from the philosophy that if change seems to be happening, it makes sense to go with what is working and stay out of the way. The second reason that no competing experience was suggested was that the therapist was not ready, because there had not been a goal established or an indication of improvement discussed.

Before suggesting that Hal consider the difficulties inherent in changing his situation, the therapist followed up his first session question regarding what an indication of change would be. Hal responded that he had thought more about the question and decided that when he could go to bed at night without everything "boiling over" for a couple hours, he would know that he was on the right track and getting better.

Excerpt Seven

T: There's something I want to ask you to do. I'd like to ask you to sit down for 30 minutes and consider the disadvantages of you starting to feel better about yourself and what roadblocks would arise. Or if you continue to move or to make a little more progress, what would be the repercussions of that. You've been a loser and depressed a long time and for good reasons—and now you are beginning to take some steps, and the obstacles that have always been there will appear or resurface to hold you back or shoot you down like they have before. I'd like for you to think about what those obstacles are and what other possible disadvantages or hindrances will block your way to feeling better about yourself. I know that's abstract, I can't make it concrete, because I want to think about it more also. But if you limit yourself to the logical and to the reasonable, you probably won't think of very many things. So you have to let your mind run kind of wild and think about it. It sounds kind of silly—what disadvantages would there be if I felt better or what obstacles will appear. But I tend to think that there would at least be implications in your family. The obvious person who comes to mind is your father, but I want to think about that some more. Does it make sense?

C: Yes, I know what you mean. I've started in the right direction before only to fall right on my face again. O.K.

T: I also want to pursue the sleep thing too, O.K.?

C: O.K.

Commentary

The suggestion continued validation of Hal's experience and brought attention to the evolving connection among Hal's dissatisfaction with his dad's control, his job, and his depression. In session three, the therapist is open to any new topics that Hal initiates, but also pursues Hal's thoughts regarding the suggestion, as well as the sleep topic.

SESSION THREE

Excerpt Eight

T: I got something from the Bureau of Vocational Rehabilitation (BVR) about you.

C: I went to see them about going back to school and getting some training, and they wanted to know who I was seeing, who I had seen about my learning disability and everything.

T: How is it going?

C: It's been about the same, highs and lows, ups and downs. During the week, it's low.

T: Do you think it's because you're working during the week?

C: It could be. During the week a lot of times I feel like I'm accomplishing absolutely nothing.

T: Accomplishing toward what goal?

C: A more independent self. I'm in the same job, the same routine, and going nowhere fast.

T: You're kind of confronted with that fact every day when you go to work and nothing happens.

C: Right.

T: How's your sleep been?

C: The same, 3 or 4 hours a night. Maximum 4 hours a night.

Commentary

Hal had taken more action. He had applied for aid from BVR to go to tech school even though he knew his father disapproved and might withdraw his support. The theme of the exception to the depression arose again, and was more clearly articulated by Hal as being related to not accomplishing anything toward his goal of independence. The therapist did not pursue it, but it seems safe to assume that Hal was implying independence from his father. Once again, the momentum seemed to be there, and the therapist wanted to ride and empower that momentum. Note in the discussion that follows how Hal's resolve and confidence build to a crescendo.

Excerpt Nine

T: O.K. I want to get back to that and find out more information about your sleep. But before I do that, I wanted to ask you if you've considered the disadvantages or dangers of being able to feel better and the obstacles that could arise that have undercut you before?

C: The major obstacle is my father.

T: O.K., let's talk about your father. I guess the major implication of your starting to feel better and being more self confident, and being more successful financially—all the way around, jobwise, any way you want to slice it—I think that would be a real jolt to your old man in a lot of ways. He has this way of looking at you that he's looked at you your whole life—a lot more than 8 years—and you've frankly, been a loser in his eyes. I think success may shake him up pretty significantly, and he's probably used to you not doing so well, and it may shake him up more than you want to if you do real well, especially in a non-white-collar job.

C: I don't want to cut the bonds between us, but at the same time, I want to break off financial bonds too, so we can get on with our life as I see it should be getting on—Rene and I. At the same time, he has to be shaken up a little bit—I'm not his puppet. Sometimes I feel like that's what he needs—a good jolt.

T: You'd kind of like to deliver that, huh?

C: Sometimes. Well, to get out from under his thumb, because ever since I can remember, he's been trying to pull punches on me, and when I did go to college, he'd say, "I don't think you should go into business, I think you should go into accounting." And when the next quarter came around, there'd be accounting on my list, because I was still a minor, and it wouldn't come off on my list of classes. So there are times he does need a good jolt, he needs to be told that I am not there for him to run my life.

T: Even though he's done it all your life.

C: He's almost like a dictator. I hate to say that about him, but he is. He likes to tell you where to go and how to do it, even though he's never done it that way. He's always done exactly the opposite of what he tells everybody else to do. So he does need a jolt, he needs to be told—maybe not in words, but in actions.

T: That's a good point, because I think talk is fairly cheap and actions—the old cliche—actions speak louder than words—and they sure do. That's why I think you getting better and being more clear about where you're going and making decisions independently of him would be quite a shock to him.

C: It might be a shock in the beginning, but I think in the end it would be a positive.

T: You think he could adjust.

C: Um huh. Deep down, he's a good man, he just wants the best for his kids. But the way he does it leaves a lot to be desired.

T: He does it by being a dictator, but he sees himself as being a benevolent dictator. But a dictator's a dictator.

C: All the way around, any way you look at it.

T: Even if they have the best intentions, they're still dictators. Sometimes the only way to get rid of a dictator is to do a coup, and that's essentially what you would be doing by getting better. You would be dethroning the dictator.

C: Get him out as the king of my life and put myself in there.

T: I just think that would be a fairly dramatic thing to do and one that he won't adjust to very well, and it would be a tremendous shock to him.

C: Well, like I say, it has to be done. The shock may last a year or two, but once it's happened, he'll realize there's no turning back. When he sits down and sees where I'm going with my life, and that he's not going to be there for the next 30 or 40 years, he's not going to be there all that time, he *has* to realize that. He may not realize it now, but in the long run he has to realize it. That's why I have to get through to him, and that's why I'm working and trying to get better, trying to improve my life.

T: Well, I guess the other one that comes to my mind—and again, just like all of them—the one about your dad makes a lot of sense to me, but this one may or may not make sense to you—but it made some sense to me as I thought about it. It's kind of a touchy area in some ways. You have had a lot of failures and a lot of troubles in your life. You were dealt a raw deal to begin with and didn't even know it and wound up devaluating yourself as a worthless kind of a person for a long time, not knowing that you had a learning disability. If you'd known those things early on, you probably would have developed a sense of competency along the way, hopefully as your son will do now. You didn't know all that, so you were kind of dealt a raw deal and had to deal with all these things. How you wound up dealing with them, I think, is, "I'm no good, I must be a lazy bum, people are right." I think over the years you did that pretty well, and, as a result of that, you were set up in losing situations time and time again. You essentially had some failures, like we talked about before. Well, the one thing about your current state, say your emotional state, and your current state of thinking about yourself—your self esteem, self confidence—is that in many ways I see that protecting you from further falls, from further losing propositions, from maybe even a deeper depression, because if you don't get better, if you don't start feeling better, you probably won't move ahead and do anything that's all that risky. You know, when you move forward and do different things, you're taking a big risk. A lot of people choose not to move forward because the risk of the fall that they'll take if it doesn't work is more of a risk or more of a disadvantage than staying the way they currently are. And that makes a lot of sense. I don't think those people are bad people, or lazy, or stupid, or anything else. I think that unconsciously they're keeping themselves together in that they're very concerned about what making a change will bring about and think that the change it brings about may be worse than what they have now. Does that make any sense?

C: Yes. What you're saying is you know where you're at, and you're trying to make the best of where you're at right then and there. But if you step out into unknown territory—fear of the unknown. You don't know where you're going, you don't know what path to take in that unmapped area. It could be worse than you have it now.

T: That's it exactly, and I think we protect ourselves from those things, and I think that protection against failure is an obstacle also, although it looks like you're really plodding forward fast in a lot of ways . . it doesn't seem to be an obstacle.

C: Time's running out. I'm 31 and to be able to get a good job, I have to get the schooling in. So to be able to get a good job and have a good retirement 30 years from now, I've got to start doing things now.

T: I guess I would agree with that. Can you think of any other disadvantages or dangers for you to start feeling better and more confident about yourself?

C: It's just shaky ground. Maybe shock my brother and sisters.

T: It would shake them up too?

C: Um huh. 'Cause I know they've called me a loser for a long time too.

T: They all have a pretty solid image of you being a loser in their minds.

C: But to give them a good jolt would be nice.

T: So you're probably going to give a right cross to everybody in your family.

C: I won't say it would be fun, but it would shake them up. Just to be able to give that little shock right now, that would feel good. To let them know I'm not what everybody thinks I am—I'm a lot better.

T: That sounds like a pretty confident statement.

C: I have to get that way. I've been so low for so long, I have to go up, I can't come down. If I go down any further, it's 6 feet under. That's the way I've seen things, and that's why I'm starting to get help, that's why I need to get help. Because of my son—I don't want him to start off on a bad footing, I want to be there to help him get that good footing. If I'm not there, I don't think he would.

T: Well I'll tell you, you are really going to shake some people up if you keep talking confidently and doing some things. They're going to do everything they can to get you back in your place. I think that's a major obstacle too. People don't like things to change.

C: My sister wouldn't.

T: I guess I'm thinking more of your father and your brother, perhaps.

C: They need that shock.

T: They'll try to pull the rug out from under you by being negative to everything you say that may even resemble being a self-confident statement.

C: In his own way, my dad's always throwing it up.

T: Somehow that doesn't surprise me a whole lot.

C: When I suggested something about going back to school, he starts picking negatively about it.

T: "You're too old for that."

C: Too old for it—How are you going to live? How's your family going to live? Why don't you go to real college?

T: You have other responsibilities, just accept your lot in life.

C: Exactly. But then again, he wants me to get on the base, and you can guess what field.

T: In accounting.

C: Of course!

T: That way you'll be right in your cubby hole, right where you belong. You'll be making a little bit more money and he'll feel like he's been benevolent.

C: He's an accountant, so that's where his son should be. The old school, like I said.

T: Like father, like son, no matter whether the son fits or not.

C: A farmer's son is a farmer, a blacksmith's son is a blacksmith, and so on down the line. I guess his son should be an accountant, no matter whether his son wants to be or not. So it's just come down to that—it's starting to be a fight—I've got to learn how to do it. Start to stand up for my own rights, because I haven't done it.

T: That's risky, you have a better reason not to. Alienating family is a good reason not to. Being defeated is a good reason not to. Standing up for your rights and then getting slaughtered when you do it is a good reason not to do it. He's still going to slice you up, and he's good at undercutting you, and he's been doing it for the last 30 years. He's going to continue to be able to do that whether you stand up or not. And you hit the nail on the head, the way you're going to do it will be behaviorally, not verbally. Maybe the verbally will come after that, after the impression has been made in the behavioral way. But I think he will undercut you—I think other people will, which will make it doubly hard for you to be able to do anything.

C: I know my brother will, there's no doubt about it. I *know* my brother will. When I started going back to school through the company, my sister was on my side—no problem, no thinking about it. She thought it was great I was trying to get an education that way. So I have no doubt where she will be. My wife will be behind me 100%, no doubt about it.

T: But the undercutters, though . . .

C: My dad and my brother—that's it.

T: That's going to be tough to get around because you're dad, I'm sure, is a pro at it by this point in your life.

C: I'm sure he's got it down to a science, I'm sure he has.

T: And I think that affects your self-esteem—it's going to take the wind out of your sails.

C: It's just—all my life I've been taught about the other person. How's the other person going to feel if you do this. And about the last year I've started to think, "When's people going to start thinking about me?" The other person's not thinking about me when they say that. You're not thinking about me when you say that, or do this or do that. That's what's getting to me now—it's 30 years of thinking about everybody else, now it's my turn. I have to start thinking about me now, otherwise there is no more me. I'm just everybody else.

T: Well, changing that's going to go over like a

C: A lead balloon.

T: A lead balloon—you bet. People get used to having others consider their needs before their own. You're going to be told how inconsiderate and selfish you are.

C: At this point, I don't care. If I can give some people a jolt, if I can teach a few people a lesson, that will make it all worthwhile. I've got to have some successes. I've got to start succeeding now.

Commentary

The conversation has now shifted from a description of Hal as a depressed loser in session one to a person ready to stand up for his own choices and prepared to have successes in life regardless of the protestations of others and the encumbrances of his father's disapproval. An evolution of meaning occurred in which the depression was no longer solely connected to Hal being a loser, but also to his dissatisfying job and his father's dictatorship. Note how the dialogue unfolded to the point where Hal replaced his own invalidation (recall session one) with strong statements of self-validation (e.g., I'm better than they think I am).

The therapist was now ready to pursue the sleep problem that Hal had indicated at the end of session two would be a sign that his depression was improving. Hal reported that he spent a couple of hours at bedtime thinking things over, reviewing what had happened during the day, and often gave himself a hard time about his lack of progress in achieving independence. Hal said that everything "boiled over" at bedtime, usually resulting in only a few hours of fitful sleep.

The therapist wanted to pull together several themes that had emerged from the therapeutic conversation in the competing experience. In many ways, the competing experience was designed to merely continue the shift in meaning that was already occurring and to reinforce the connections Hal was making regarding his father, his job, and the exception he noted that his depression generally happened during the week.

The competing experience was also designed to provide another way of interrupting Hal's solution attempts of ignoring the depression, singing his way through it, and boiling it all over at bedtime in a way that was generally unproductive. Hal's primary emphasis in his description of both the depression and his sleeping troubles were cognitive, although not exclusively. It was Hal's presentation of the indication of improvement and the discussion of the review process that he undertook at bedtime that directed the therapist toward a more cognitive focus.

The delivery of the competing experience came on the tail of a discussion about the disadvantages of change that validated Hal's reasons for not already changing and justified Hal's difficulties to date in attempting to usurp his father's control and make a more satisfactory life for himself. That discussion placed Hal in the position of experiencing the therapist's suggestion as an out-of-session extension of a context that validated both Hal's desire for change and his difficulties in accomplishing it.

Excerpt Ten

T: I wanted to make a suggestion for you to consider. One way of looking at the process you go through each night that ultimately winds up in you staying awake half the night is that you are going over the events of the day and, in essence, evaluating yourself—things begin boiling over in your mind—all this stuff you're experiencing, your dad's control, the unsatisfactory job, your learning disability, the tech school, etc. starts demanding "airtime" or for you to give your situation undivided attention. While it certainly is frustrating, it may be useful as well if it is focused toward sorting all this stuff out. I was thinking that you could take charge of this review process, accepting that it is going to happen anyway, and structure it in a way that you can get through it more quickly and get to sleep more quickly. Also, the new structure may give some different information about your depression. Am I making any sense?

C: Yes, like since I'm doing it anyway, why not make the best of it—but what structure are you talking about?

T: What I was thinking was that right before you go to bed tonight, rate the level of depression that you think or predict you will experience tomorrow, on a scale of 10 to 1, where 10 is least depressed and 1 is most depressed. Then tomorrow night at bedtime, rate your actual level of depression on the same scale. Once you have the two numbers, the predicted rate and the actual rate, review the events of the day and try to make sense of any discrepancies. For example, if you predicted a 3 or a pretty lousy day, and you actually experienced a 6 or a not-so-bad day, then you would go over the day and try to figure what made the difference. Am I sounding like an idiot or does this seem reasonable?

C: No, I understand. I'm supposed to compare the two numbers and figure out why they're different.

Commentary

The de Shazer et al. (1986) depression task interrupted Hal's current solutions, matched his primary cognitive emphasis, and was delivered in a context of validation. The competing experience emerged from and reinforced significant aspects of the interview process so that the quest for change opportunities would extend to between sessions as well. Hal's noted exception, as well as his connections between his depression and his father and job, could be further highlighted by the depression task, although such an outcome could not be predicted. The therapist's task in the next session was to approach Hal and his out-of-session experience with a sense of natural curiosity, remaining open to Hal's input and any new information that might arise.

SESSION FOUR

Excerpt Eleven

T: It's been a while since you were here, I think 4 weeks, so how is it going?

C: Well, a lot of things have happened. You're not going to believe all this. First, I got canned at the loan company right after I was here last. They had a reduction in force layoff, which I was kind of expecting for some time. So I had the time and followed up with BVR and found out they rejected my application for aid to go to school. They said they didn't consider my learning disability to be the kind of disability that they gave aid for to return people to school. I decided to apply to tech school anyway, because I found out that I could get loans through them—then the shit really hit the fan. My dad blew up and withdrew financial support. It was a very big deal, but it's not going to change my mind, I'm going to tech school anyway.

T: This is too much.

C: Yeah [laughing], I know.

T: No, really, I mean this is mindboggling. This is quite a disheartening turn of events, the layoff, the BVR rejection, and your dad cutting you off. You already experienced an essentially lifelong pattern of being a loser, which resulted in a predictable depression, and now, more garbage to deal with on top of all that. But, honestly, I'm confused—you're telling me that you responded to losing your job, being rejected by BVR, and being cut off by dad by enrolling in technical school? This doesn't seem to add up or fit with all that's happened. You don't seem defeated by it all.

C: Well, I've done a lot of thinking in the past few weeks—about my life and about our sessions—and I have come to the conclusion that the only way I can start having some successes is to start doing what I think is important. You know that depression rating at bedtime thing? Well, the more I thought of the events of the day, the more the fog cleared, and the more I saw that I will never be happy while I'm working a loser job and under the dictatorship of my dad.

T: Let me make sure I'm getting this. You're saying that you responded to these horrendous circumstances by telling yourself you'd never be happy in your current situation and *that* made you feel better?

C: Ha, ha. No, not exactly. I had some real shitty days because of losing the job and worrying about money and all, but I resolved that I was going to do something about my loser lifestyle, because I was going to be depressed until I did. So, I enrolled in tech school, and I'm on my way. Funny too, I'm sleeping better, except when I'm so excited about thinking of tech school.

T: I'm glad you're sleeping better, and I'm understanding better, but I'm still somewhat amazed how you were able to overcome feeling depressed and even suicidal again when the ax fell, and your dad pulled his stunt.

C: I decided that now I was going to take charge of my life and call the shots, not my dad. I've always wanted to be a computer repairman but never wanted to deal with dad, who always wanted me to be just like him and go to regular college.

T: That was a tough decision, based on the unfairness of your life and the obstacle of your father's disapproval.

C: I had to do it. I've just decided that life isn't going to defeat me any longer.

Commentary

A competing experience was suggested to Hal within a context that validated both his desire to change and his difficulties in doing so. The intervention was also designed to pull together and highlight several different themes that had evolved in the therapeutic conversation. Once Hal reported the new information regarding losing his job and the rest, and his response of enrolling in tech school, the therapist recognized that a shift in meaning had occurred. The therapeutic focus then moved to a promotion of a therapeutic dialogue designed to expand and further empower the new meaning being ascribed by Hal. The serendipitous event of being laid off and the competing experience seemed to set the context for Hal to revise his meaning from accepting a loser's lifestyle to taking definitive action to improve his situation. The therapist punctuated the shift in meaning by asking questions that encouraged Hal to articulate the changes that he was experiencing. Further change was therefore empowered through the client's own positive self-ascriptions without the therapist taking responsibility for the change. The culmination of the empowering client-ascribed meaning sequence and Hal taking responsibility is best illustrated by his comment, "I just plain decided that I was not going to let life defeat me anymore."

The rest of the session was spent discussing the tech school and the pitfalls associated with being a student. Another appointment was set for 6 weeks.

SESSION FIVE

Excerpt Twelve

T: You look different. [Client had grown a beard.]

C: I'm in my grubbies, I'm a student.

T: How is it going?

C: Everything is going O.K. I'm getting into the swing of things. I'm getting the basics. It's going to be fun. I think I'm going to pull through. It looks good.

T: It looks good?

C: It looks real good. I got a pat on the back from my instructor.

T: Already.

C: Already. We got our kits for our projects, and we were going through some of our inventory pieces and one capacitor was not listed on the inventory sheet. No one else could find it, but I identified it. The instructor asked me if I had taken electronics before. I said, "No," and he said, "How did you know that?" I said, "Instinct," and he said, "Go with your instinct. If your instinct is that good, you have the talent." So when I was walking away, I was 5 feet off the ground.

T: That's great!

C: Even Dad is helping out again. He doesn't like this [pointing to his beard]. He doesn't like the jeans either, but he came around and started helping financially again.

T: That's an amazing turnaround for him, but it's also quite a turnaround for you.

C: I know . . . it all hit at the same time—I'm kind of spinning—the loan company, the tech school, it was just . . . when I left the loan company it was just like the flood gates were open. It was amazing, it was like the loan company was the band and when that broke, everything else started coming in. It was like the loan company was the depression. When I got rid of the loan company, I got rid of the depression. At that point, I had been working there for 3 years and had depression for 5 years before that. I don't know, I feel better, I feel like things are finally going my way, I'm finally starting to accomplish things. I know I can get through tech school. In my gut, I know it's going to happen, I just feel that way. I've finally found my talent—where I'm supposed to be in the world. I finally found my niche.

T: Well, you've known it for a long time, but now . . .

C: I'm proving it—this is neat, it's fun.

T: It's fun having successful experiences for a change.

C: This is fun, quite a high.

Commentary

Again, the dialogue is best characterized by the encouragement of the client to articulate further the shift in meaning he has experienced. The therapist made several passes, which led to the following sequence.

Excerpt Thirteen

C: When I got rid of the loan company, I felt better. You know, I was expecting it—the canning.

T: Right, you suspected that early on.

C: When it came, I wasn't depressed.

T: I know, it seemed like you were—"I knew this was going to happen and I have my plans"—it was pretty amazing in a lot of ways.

C: And my dad was pulling back my support.

T: I'm still amazed at that process. When things were the absolute worst for you, you did not have a defeated attitude—there was something weirdly different about that.

C: I was amazed.

T: I was too. There was something about you that was different—the end of your job, BVR turning you down, your dad withdrawing support—everything went down the tubes at once. And you had the attitude that things were going to work out because, "I'm going to make it work"—and I tried to figure out why in the hell you weren't in the pits with depression.

C: It was like something clicked—I don't know if you felt it—something clicked in me. I couldn't let it defeat me—if I let it defeat me, that was it, that was the end of my life, because from then on out, my dad was going to run my life. I couldn't let it defeat me. It was no longer going to be me in this body, but me and him.

T: But after your history, how in the world did this happen? Always before these kinds of things would have been another nail in your coffin, another failure.

C: I'm amazed at it myself.

T: Sounds like magic.

C: You're right, like magic. I don't know where it came from—like some *inner strength kicked in*, something I've been looking for all this time.

T: Right when you needed it the most, you were able to find this inner strength and pull it out.

C: Right. Now that I'm here, now that I know what's going on, I'm riding high because I'm in charge, not my wife, not my mother, not my *dad*, I'm in charge. It's a good feeling. I enjoy where I am right now. I have no doubt I'll graduate from school and get the job I want. I can't let it get back to where it was. I think I finally found that inner strength where it wasn't. I value myself—not like 4 or 5 months ago. I questioned everything about me. I was a total loser. But now I feel better about myself, especially in class where I know what's going on.

T: I'm glad you found your inner strength . . . well, what do you want to do about continuing therapy?

C: No, I'm ready to quit. I feel guilty about sitting here.

T: You feel guilty about not studying—that's fine.

C: That's a kicker in itself. I feel guilty about not being able to study. Ha!

T: Ha, ha.

C: Before it was always, "What's the use in studying when I'll just fail anyway."

T: I've enjoyed working with you.

C: It's been real helpful—just getting all the years off my back—this helped *me find my inner strength.*

Commentary

This session climaxed when Hal commented that he had found his inner strength and had overcome his loser lifestyle. Hal was on a roll of positive self-ascriptions and was taking responsibility for the changes he was making. The therapist moved to the question regarding termination, given Hal's indicator for change had been met (sleep problem). and the depression was significantly improved. Hal's response was another indication of his improvement—he felt guilty about taking the time from studying! Being in the world had become far more important than being in therapy.

Hal's final statement illustrates what we consider to be a perfect ending to therapy. He commented that therapy *helped* him find *his* inner strength. Rather than repairing any deficits or curing any disorders, therapy assisted Hal to utilize the resources he always possessed, but had difficulty in accessing.

DISCUSSION

The case of Hal summarizes all the pieces of information discussed in this book and is an excellent example of the incredible propensity that people have to make rapid meaningful changes with minimal therapeutic intervention. Recall that Hal was referred by his company's EAP because his problem could not be addressed in the limited three to five sessions that the EAP could provide. It's interesting to note that Hal's depression was not only improved, but his life took an entirely different direction in the confines of just five sessions. This is not a testament to our approach, as much as it is a confirmation of the powerful capacity of individuals to find their "inner strength" in remarkably short periods of time. If one holds the assumption that certain problems or client presentations cannot be adequately dealt with in short periods of time or that meaningful change cannot occur rapidly, then it is quite likely that those assumptions will prove accurate.

The therapist embraced a process-constructive theoretical frame-work and held a different set of assumptions in his work with Hal. As an overall guiding theory, the interaction between Hal and the therapist was viewed as a "system" involving an ongoing exchange of meaning that inevitably and continually revises as variability or new information is added by the therapist or client. The therapist assumed from his constructivist theoretical base that Hal had generated a meaning system that he was a loser and that everything he did only confirmed that conclusion. Hal's organization of his perceptions and experiences was accepted by the therapist as the theory from which he operated. In other words, Hal's content-rich and value-laden description of his life experience, his informal theory of the depression, took precedence over any content-based formal theory of the therapist.

The therapist's process-based description of Hal's depression placed it in the context of all the failures Hal had experienced (a series of incidental events), which reinforced his "loser" meaning system, and in the context of a developmental struggle to escape from his father's financial control. Hal's depression, from a process view, was also seen as exacerbated by Hal's and others' attempts at solution.

Seeing Hal's depression problem as interactional in nature and working from Hal's presented content, the therapist operationalized empathy, respect, and genuineness by validating Hal's experience of his life. Hal seemed to interpret the relationship as empathic, respectful, and genuine, given his comments about the relationship: "Someone understands, talking about this cleared the fog, released the pressure, helped me get the years off my back, etc." The therapist validated not only Hal's experience of being a loser, but also his struggles with changing his situation. A positive alliance was fostered by the agreement of goals (sleep indicator) and tasks (depression rating suggestion) of therapy.

Exploring and unfolding Hal's perception and experience led to an emergence of Hal's recognition of his dissatisfaction with his job and his financial dependence on his father. The conversational recreation of Hal's experience allowed an evolution of meaning to occur that shifted Hal's "loser" meaning to a confident person ready to pursue a different career path, even though his father disapproved.

The competing experience (depression rating) extended the validation context into Hal's social environment and reinforced the connections Hal was making during session. Hal continued to ascribe self-empowering meaning that enabled him to take significant actions to address his job and father dissatisfactions. The therapy process only set the context for Hal to find his "inner strength" and risk the meaning revision necessary for problem improvement.

8   Marital Case Study: "Mr. Spock"

THIS chapter presents excerpts from each session of a marital case and provides commentary explaining the therapeutic process. This case illustrates the additional challenges and opportunities that occur when more than one person is involved in therapy. Recall from Chapter 4 that the couple is interviewed together and separately to enable three different sets of opportunities to promote meaningful change. The marital problem(s) may be altered by either person initiating a change in the problematic patterns of interaction, or by the couple acting together to address a particular concern.

Steven and Mary Ann were referred to marital therapy by their pastor. They were in their early 30s, had been married 7 years, and had two children, ages 1 and 2. The pastor told the therapist that Steven was ambivalent about staying in the marriage and that Mary Ann was confused about what to do about it.

SESSION ONE

Excerpt One

T: What brings you here to see me today?

S: Well, lots of things, but mainly because I'm not sure if I love Mary Ann anymore, and I don't know if I want to stay married.

T: Mary Ann, what brings you here?

M: I'm trying to understand what Steven is so upset about so I can work on saving our marriage—but I don't know what to do—I can't figure out why he is giving me a hard time.

S: I don't know what there is to figure out. You don't, or can't meet my emotional needs; and I'm not sure I can stay with someone for the rest of my life who can't provide me with the kind of emotional intimacy that I want from a relationship [voice rising].

M: Well, maybe if you weren't so cold and critical and spent a little time helping me with the kids, I would be able to give you whatever it is you're talking about [voice trembling, starting to cry].

Commentary

After a period of silence, the therapist decided to separate the couple because it seemed as if the tension was inhibiting an open exchange about the problem. The therapist wanted to pursue with each person the issue or problem that needed to be addressed for both to experience a successful outcome. Steven quickly volunteered to go first.

Excerpt Two

S: I just don't think I have any feelings for Mary Ann anymore. From the beginning of the marriage, I've been the one that gives more to the relationship, and I'm tired of giving without receiving. I'm not like most guys. I really enjoy and crave emotional intimacy. She is just not what I want anymore.

T: And how would you like her to be?

S: I'd like her to just be a warm, caring human being. I want an enthusiastic woman who is deeply in love with me and is not afraid to show it. I want her to wrap her arms around my neck, look me in the eyes for several seconds, and say, "I love you." I want to go for an intimate stroll through a park, holding each other as if everything around us was not even there. I want her to appreciate my words of intimacy and my affectionate advances. I want her to share her thoughts and feelings throughout the day and be interested in my thoughts and feelings.

T: Sounds like you're feeling real deprived, and maybe a little angry at Mary Ann for not giving you what you want.

S: That's exactly it. I guess the rest of the problem is that we just don't connect anymore—we never talk about the relationship, only small talk. Mary Ann never talks about feelings, and there's no emotional closeness between us. I guess the main thing is that we just don't communicate about the relationship at a feeling level. Mary Ann seems just committed to the children, especially since our second child was born. She never has anything left for anything or anyone else.

T: You're feeling left out and neglected.

S: Yes, big time, but it's more than that because I don't think Mary Ann is capable of giving me what I want. She is just not a deep person. She is just not sensitive to feelings in general, her own or mine.

T: How is she insensitive to your feelings?

S: 'How isn't she,' would be a better question. No matter how bad my day is or how much I am struggling with the pressures of my life, she never, I mean never, picks up on it. She just goes on about her routine and is completely out of touch with my feelings. Mary Ann is not emotionally supportive.

T: So is it safe to say that you are questioning your feelings for Mary Ann because of her inability to communicate about your relationship and her insensitivity to your feelings?

S: Yes. I used to think that she didn't care, but now I think Mary Ann is incapable of expressing feelings or being sensitive to mine. As you know, some people are like that.

T: Uh huh. How do you know that your wife is one of those people?

S: Mary Ann is from a dysfunctional family. I've discussed this with my brother, who is a therapist at an alcohol treatment center, and he said that Mary Ann's family sounds real dysfunctional to him, even though both her parents are not alcoholics. My brother said that the family seemed emotionally cut off from each other and that Mary Ann probably grew up in a "don't talk, don't trust, don't feel" family of origin. Her family is real weird. They never argue or show affection that I've ever seen. My brother also said that Mary Ann would always have an emotional dysfunction unless she got into therapy or worked a 12-step program in an adult children of alcoholics group (ACOA). He talked to her about it and recommended that Mary Ann start attending ACOA groups, but she said that she didn't see the relevance. Here my brother was trying to help her see her dysfunction, and she ignored it just like all the times I've told her there was something wrong about her, because she never is sensitive enough to pick up signals from me that I need support. She's in denial.

T: So you have tried to address this problem with Mary Ann?

S: I've tried until I'm blue in the face. I've explained to her what I need, I've pointed out to her when she isn't being supportive, and I've really tried to encourage her to express her feelings about things—she is just a cold fish—she needs help and unless she gets it, I'm not staying around.

T: Sounds like you've tried a lot. Have you tried anything else?

S: I tried confronting her like my brother suggested, but that never seems to go anywhere. Now I'm just trying to detach and stay the hell away from her. It's her responsibility anyway. I guess sometimes my hostility comes through too, but basically that's all I've been doing lately.

T: What would be an indication to you that things were beginning to move in the right direction? What would be a sign that Mary Ann was starting to communicate more at a feeling level and starting to become more sensitive to your feelings?

S: Mary Ann would initiate a conversation about how she felt about something other than the kids, and would be interested in how I felt as well.

T: Given that Mary Ann seems to be unable to meet you at your level, or even knows what your level is, it's no wonder you're having mixed feelings and questioning your love for her. Well, I'd better talk to her now. [Steven leaves, and the therapist invites Mary Ann to join him.]

T: So, Mary Ann, what do you think is going on here?

M: You know, I really don't know what he is so upset over. I do know that I don't seem to do anything right. I'm trying to understand what he wants, but it's hard with all his pressuring and putting me down. Every time I turn around, Steven points out to me another chance I missed to be supportive or how my time with him is just as important as my time with the kids. He's so possessive of my time. But maybe he is right, maybe it is my fault, because I get so overwhelmed with all the stuff I have to do just taking care of two little kids.

T: Really. I just have one infant son, and it seems like all we do is work to take care of him—bottles, laundry, diapers—it's never-ending, and nothing else seems to ever get done.

M: Exactly. I'm doing something all the time, and when I finally get done, I'm so exhausted that I just pass out. Maybe if I felt better at night I could give Steven the attention that he wants and figure out how to "communicate," his favorite word, with him. But he expects so much. He wants me to handle the kids all day, do my job—I do telephone soliciting for an auto club—and then be waiting at home for him with a candlelight dinner and a rose in my teeth. And somehow I'm supposed to figure out if he is in a good mood or not. He says that I'm not in touch. Maybe he is right, but I try.

T: Sounds like maybe Steven is not so "in touch" with the difficulty inherent in taking care of two small children.

M: That's for sure. When he gets home, he does nothing to help me with dinner or the kids. He just sits in front of the TV or his pet computer. That reminds me . . . this will give you an idea of what he expects from me. Steven really wanted a laser printer for his birthday. He hinted at it several times, so I went out and bought one. When I gave it to him, he said that it would have been nice if I would have figured it out without him having to hint so strongly . . . that if I would have really been connected to him I would have realized how important the computer is to him and would have known that a laser printer would please him. We went out to dinner for his birthday; I planned the whole thing, just like he likes for me to—and he wound up giving me a hard time because I didn't have a glass of wine, and I wasn't being romantic enough.

T: No matter what you did, it didn't quite measure up to what Steven wanted. Pretty maddening.

M: Really, sometimes I get so mad at him, but he's so convincing. He can talk me into anything. Maybe he is right. Maybe I'm not capable of real emotion because of my upbringing. My parents never really said much to each other or to the kids. I try to talk to Steven, but when I do, he tells me what I am saying is trivial or I'm talking on the surface and not really discussing my deep feelings. If I don't say anything, then he criticizes me about that.

T: You're literally damned if you do and damned if you don't. Steven criticizes you?

M: Yes, a lot. He calls me an emotionless robot, says I'm in denial, and says I'm too caught up in practical things. Sometimes he calls me Mr. Spock. He puts me down about other things too. When I argue back, he just criticizes me more. Steven is a great arguer. I always lose, he is always in control.

T: What do you do when Steven puts you down or criticizes you for something?

M: Like I said, I argue back, but he's a lot better at it, and he always can turn things around to be my fault no matter what it is. I've tried explaining to him my reasons for whatever it is I did or didn't do, but he never accepts my reasons, but usually criticizes my reasons too. Sometimes I cry.

T: Does that make him back off?

M: No, he usually says that at least I can cry, at least I'm capable of some emotional response.

T: Have you tried anything else?

M: I read an assertiveness book and tried a couple of things, but Steven is a lot better talker than I am, and he can twist things around so quickly I don't know whether I'm coming or going. I really don't know what to do. I'm just very confused.

T: No wonder you're confused. Look at all the ways you have tried to meet Steven's needs only to be met with rejection, criticism, and withdrawal. You try to do something he wants, but he finds something wrong with it. You try to talk to him, but you don't do it in the right way. On top of all that, while he is being demanding of your emotional support, it doesn't appear that he gives much of his own, either emotionally, or in terms of helping around the house.

M: I have tried to make him happy.

T: What would be an indication to you that things were getting a little better between you and Steven?

M: Well, I guess that I would know that Steven still cared for me if he would help a little more without being asked and stop criticizing me so much. He has withdrawn so much, I really don't think he loves me anymore. If he didn't criticize me and didn't pressure me so much about "connecting," I think everything would be better.

T: I'd like to take a little break now, and collect my thoughts. I'll come to the waiting room in about 10 minutes.

Commentary

The therapist believed that he had a good initial pass at what each person saw as the problem, solutions they had tried, and what they were looking for from therapy. Questions aimed at what Steven's feelings of ambivalence were about, and how his marriage was troubled led to Steven defining the problem as Mary Ann's "inability to communicate about the relationship and her insensitivity to his feelings." Steven believed that Mary Ann suffered from an emotional deficit resulting from her experiences in her family of origin.

When asked what an indication would be that things were beginning to turn in the right direction, Steven said that Mary Ann would be willing to discuss the relationship and would openly share her feelings, as well as attempt to understand his feelings. Steven's attempts to address the lack of communication and insensitivity to his feelings were characterized by open expression of his concerns, followed by criticism of Mary Ann's inadequate response, and finally followed by avoidance of her and withdrawal from household and childcare responsibilities.

Mary Ann was resentful of Steven's persistent discontent and reported that it seemed as if she couldn't do anything right. In her view, Steven expected her to handle the kids all day and be waiting for him with open arms *and* legs when he arrived home. Mary Ann noted a communication problem, but described the problem as his attacks and criticisms of her. Mary Ann said that she was beginning to believe that there was something wrong with her.

Mary Ann reported that Steven also criticized other things, and she felt intimidated by him in conversations because he always seemed to be in control. She noted that if Steven would help her with the house or kids without being asked, it would also be an indication of improvement. Mary Ann's solutions included telling Steven that she didn't like being criticized, defending and justifying her behavior, and crying. She had also read an assertiveness book with similar results.

The interview with Steven redefined the problem from a lack of feeling for Mary Ann, to a dissatisfaction with her communication difficulties and emotional insensitivity. Two opportunities arose from the interview: One involved the problem cycle of Steven's attempts (criticism and withdrawal) to gain communication and support from Mary Ann, and the other involved Steven's view of Mary Ann as emotionally deficient. Two avenues for change also emerged from the interview with Mary Ann: one pertaining to the problem cycle of Mary Ann's attempt (defending, justifying, etc.) to decrease Steven's criticisms, and the other involving Mary Ann's view that she didn't and couldn't understand what Steven wanted from her.

Another opportunity arose from both individuals' statements of what would constitute an indication of improvement. The therapist could pursue a homework assignment or competing experience that addressed Steven's desire for more feeling-oriented conversation and Mary Ann's wish for more help with evening responsibilities.

Recall Mary Ann's belief that she should have figured out what Steven wanted and her own invalidating comment that maybe Steven was right about her incapability of real emotion. The therapist highlighted the ways that Mary Ann had tried to provide what Steven wanted and how her attempts were largely met with rejection and withdrawal. The therapist commented that no wonder Mary Ann was at a loss for what to do.

The therapist offered validation of her experience with Steven that replaced the invalidation of his perspective (emotionless robot), as well as her own invalidation. "I should have figured this out, maybe he is right." Replacing an invalidating experience opens the possibility for rapid change. The therapist also validated Steven's experience of ambivalence about his feelings about his wife and marriage. Steven's story did not seem to carry the invalidation that characterized Mary Ann's.

In consideration of suggesting a competing experience, the therapist believed, and depended upon the fact, that Steven and Mary Ann had the resources necessary for problem resolution. What the clients wanted from therapy seemed very clear, and the therapist began a search for intervention options that might directly address Steven's desire for Mary Ann's initiation of conversation on a feeling level, and Mary Ann's request for Steven to help with evening responsibilities without being asked.

A general problem definition of marital strife and the couple's individually presented concerns of Mary Ann's emotional deficiency (Steven) and Steven's criticisms (Mary Ann) yielded several possible intervention options. Given the lack of time to explore collaboratively the best intervention fit, the therapist decided to suggest a variation on an observe assignment that would utilize their indications for improvement. The suggestion of an observe competing experience (formula task) was based entirely on client-generated content and goals and was attempting to promote the conditions for the couple to initiate and notice changes in each other. The observe assignment also could bring back more information that would enable further selection of additional competing experiences.

Excerpt Three

T: Let me begin by saying that I am impressed with both of your willingness to try marital therapy. It takes a lot of courage to talk to a stranger, about problems and a lot of people, quite frankly, would just throw in the towel or live with the misery before consulting with a therapist. I believe that coming here says something about each of you that is quite positive, and it says something about your desires to save your marriage. In a lot of ways, it is not surprising your problems are occurring now, given all the changes that have happened in your lives in the past 2 years—not one kid, but two more human beings totally dependent on both of you for existence—which have turned your lives

upside down. All the additional adjustments, sacrifices, and responsibilities often take their toll on the relationship. Your marriage seems to
be in a state of transition, still adjusting to the demands of parenting,
while trying to negotiate what the new couple relationship will be . .
. I was thinking of asking you two to do something, if you are willing
to engage in an experiment that may help all three of us maybe learn
more about your relationship.

S: Sure, what?

M: [Nods head]

T: Steven, I was wondering if you would be willing to do something that
involved household chores or child care without commenting about it
to Mary Ann, and then observe how things go between you and Mary
Ann to see if your good deed had any effect at all on your relationship.

S: Yes, okay. I'm not supposed to say anything, right?

T: Right. Mary Ann, would you be willing to initiate a conversation about
anything, as long as that conversation would include the expression of
your feelings about the topic and that you would inquire about
Steven's thoughts and feelings, and then observe the results that follow
between you and Steven. Also, please don't comment on the fact that
you are doing it.

M: It can be about anything I want?

T: Yes.

M: Sure.

Commentary

The homework assignment, or competing experience, was designed to
interrupt the current solution attempts of both Steven and Mary Ann by
initiating behaviors appreciably different from Steven's criticism and
avoidance, and Mary Ann's defending. The couple's indications of
improvement provided useful information for designing the assignment:
The assignment was based in client-generated content and directly
addressed the couple's reason for entering therapy. From a solution-
focused perspective (de Shazer, 1985), such an intervention sets the stage
for clients to notice exceptions to their problem that can be further
amplified by the therapeutic process.

From a meaning revision perspective, the homework assignment
included Steven's emphasis on affect and Mary Ann's on behavior such
that the task promoted an affectively and behaviorally altered experience
for the couple. The in vivo competition encouraged by the intervention

set the conditions for both individuals to revise their meanings attributed to the relationship.

The suggestion "to do something without comment and observe," given to the couple together represented a way to initiate change while simultaneously avoiding the pitfall of disconfirming either person's frame of reference. The suggestion precluded judgment about who was right or wrong, but provided a face-saving way that Mary Ann and Steven might try something different without admitting the incorrectness of their positions. By addressing each of their desires, the competing experience validated both of their subjective experiences of the marital problems.

SESSION TWO

Excerpt Four

T: How did the experiment go? Were you able to do it?

S: Well, I think it went very well. Mary Ann initiated conversations on two occasions and talked about her feelings, as well as asked me about mine.

T: What were the conversations about?

S: One was about the Gulf War, and one was about the future of our relationship. She said that she felt sad about the soldiers who had to leave their kids behind. We wound up having a long conversation about the whole thing from a lot of different angles. It was very enjoyable.

T: What was the most enjoyable part for you, Steven?

S: Well, I really liked the feeling that we were really connecting—I know Mary Ann hates that word—but I felt really good, especially the other conversation in which Mary Ann asked me where I thought the relationship would be in 5 years and she told me that she felt confident that we would still be together, that we would overcome our problems. It made me feel very hopeful.

T: How so?

S: Well, I was encouraged to see Mary Ann make an honest effort to get beyond the day-to-day routine and relate to me in a *real* fashion. I felt hope about the relationship.

T: How were you able to do it, Mary Ann?

M: Well, we had been getting along a lot better all week, and Steven helped with dinner a couple of times and with baths and bedtime at least three times. We were just a lot more involved as a couple trying to help each other be a family.

T: Great! But how were you able to initiate a conversation on such a deep level, when that had been so hard before?

M: I think mainly because I felt so much more relaxed, and I think I appreciated Steven's company a lot more. I guess I felt more like I wanted to talk to him. I've been so mad at him.

T: Steven, how were you able to pitch in with dinner and help with the kids?

S: As the week went on, and we kept getting along and talking more, it became easier and easier to help—and it did make a difference in the way the evening went. One night I came home and immediately started playing with the kids while Mary Ann made dinner. I loaded the dishwasher and gave our 2-year-old, a bath while Mary Ann took care of the baby. After bedtime is when Mary Ann started talking about the relationship. I think that one thing I learned was that working as a team with the kids seemed to help Mary Ann feel closer to me—at least that's what I felt.

T: What do you think?

M: Yes, it just seemed more like I thought family life would be.

Commentary

The therapist quickly noticed a difference in the couple's presentation in session two. Both were smiling, and the tension that characterized the first session seemed to have diminished. The therapist pursued a sequence of questions that encouraged the couple to elaborate the noted changes and continue to ascribe relationship-enhancing meanings to their successes. This interventive process of "empowering client-ascribed meaning" emphasizes the client's own positive self-ascriptions without the therapist assuming a cheerleading role. Steven's ambivalence seemed to be replaced with encouragement and hope. Mary Ann's defensiveness gave way to enjoyment of Steven's company.

Excerpt Five

The therapist separated the couple and pursued Mary Ann's presented problem with Steven's criticisms and Steven's view of Mary Ann as emotionally dysfunctional.

T: Things seem a lot better.

M: Things are great compared to before, but unfortunately, Steven still put me down a few times. It's very frustrating. I tried to rationally give him reasons, but he never accepts them, and it always ends up where I feel completely under his control. I wind up getting real defensive, which he never fails to point out, and he just continues to criticize me even more for my inability to take constructive criticism!

T: Sounds exasperating. You said you read an assertiveness book before and tried something. What happened?

M: I tried "I" statements to tell Steven how much his criticisms hurt my feelings. The same thing wound up happening. Steven said that sometimes the truth hurts and that I was trying to use what I learned in the book as a way to get out of facing the facts. Like I said, he's a better talker and can quickly turn everything around that I say. I can't think that fast, and before I know it, I've got that same old crummy feeling that he got me again. When I try to explain that to him, he acts like he doesn't know what I'm talking about. I don't have a prayer with him in any kind of discussion. He's always in control. Frankly, I think he just knows how to manipulate me.

T: Well, I thought about this criticism problem, and I wanted to bounce an idea off of you. It may sound a little off the wall and it may not fit your particular circumstance, so please feel free to tell me if it sounds too weird to try—but it is a way to handle verbal manipulation and criticism when you've already tried to directly let the other person know that you don't like it.

M: I'm all ears.

T: Given that the discussions that follow Steven's criticisms seem never to be productive, but rather result in you feeling manipulated and controlled, the strategy that I suggest that you consider is called "agree and exaggerate," that you actually respond to his criticism by agreeing with the criticism and, perhaps, even expand on it. Keep in mind that only words are involved here. You are only agreeing with words, you are not in any way changing your behavior. For example, if Steven criticizes your driving, you may respond with, "Yes, I'm a terrible driver, and I can't believe you're brave enough to ride with me." It is important that you not sound sarcastic. By doing this, you may go from a no-win to a no-lose situation. Before, when you protested or tried to defend or justify, you lost because Steven found other verbal ways to use what you said against you. If you said nothing or didn't address his criticism, he attacked you for not communicating with him. With this strategy, if you agree and Steven accepts it, the argument is over, you don't get angry and defensive, and you still handle the criticized situation however you would like. The difference is that you have exercised control over the criticism instead of it over you. If Steven disagrees with you—remember you are now accepting the criticism— he is absolving you of blame. You win again. I think that a lot of people believe that they have to win an argument or refute a criticism and prove innocence to gain control. I believe that people win when they break an old destructive pattern and decide what the new pattern will be. Some people find that it feels good not to be defensive and not to argue. It may also allow Steven to look at his criticism without being compelled to do so. Am I making any sense?

M: Oh yes. I think I can give it a try. I see how it could help me stay out of the verbal battles that Steven always wins. [Mary Ann leaves, and Steven enters.]

T: Sounds like things are better.

S: Yes, a lot better, and like I said, I'm a lot more hopeful. I'm especially hopeful that Mary Ann will address her emotional problem.

T: Sounds like, from what you told me before, that Mary Ann's family does not verbally express their feelings very freely. How do they seem otherwise?

S: Well, they seem to get along okay. I mean, they never seem mad at one another, but isn't it normal for people to be angry and fight from time to time?

T: Sure, I think so, but in some families, they just do things differently. There are a lot of ways to express feelings or communicate other than by words alone. Thinking back over your experiences with Mary Ann's parents, do you ever see them *doing* things that may represent signs of affection or caring?

S: Well, yes . . . Mary Ann's dad always helps her mom around the house. In fact, they do all kinds of things together, and I guess for each other as well.

T: So maybe, does it seem reasonable to conclude that Mary Ann grew up in an environment that in the absence of good healthy verbal expressions of feelings, that her parents tended to express themselves behaviorally rather than verbally?

S: Yes.

T: So Mary Ann may be capable of expressing her emotions behaviorally, but has difficulty doing it verbally because of her experience, or lack of it, in her family of origin.

S: That makes sense because Mary Ann has always had trouble telling me that she loved me, but she always did things for me that showed me that she did. At least she used to before our second child was born.

T: You and Mary Ann are a bit different that way. You speak different languages, and I can see how you would really become frustrated and feel hopeless in your attempts to connect with her because you are actually communicating at different levels. It may be that Mary Ann is not in fact not as deep, but rather she speaks a language that does not lend itself to an open exchange between you. Mary Ann speaks a behavioral language, and you speak a verbal language. She expresses her emotions through her behavior, while you feel most comfortable expressing your feelings verbally. But I don't think it always has to be that way. I think you can help Mary Ann learn to express herself more verbally by first speaking her language more. I think it may encourage Mary Ann to speak a more verbal language if you continue speaking her language by helping her with the kids and household stuff. By speaking her language, she may attempt to speak yours more, and some common ground can be achieved.

S: Okay. I'll keep trying, I'll speak her language, but I really would like to find some *verbal* common ground. Do you think that's possible?

T: Yes, I do. I'll give it some thought. [The couple is reunited.] Would you be willing to continue the experiment?

S: Yes, of course.

M: Uh huh.

T: Great.

Commentary

After Steven left, Mary Ann reiterated her belief that things were much better but that Steven had criticized her on a few occasions. She tried to defend herself and justify why she did things the way she did, but ultimately felt defeated and under Steven's control. Through collaborative exploration of intervention options, assertiveness training was ruled out, given Mary Ann's lack of success with previous assertive attempts. The therapist suggested that Mary Ann stop defending and justifying her actions, but rather agree with the criticisms and even exaggerate them (Duncan & Rock, 1991). The purpose would be to decrease the criticisms and allow Mary Ann to feel more in control.

In the interview with Steven, the therapist pursued the opportunity that arose from the first session regarding Mary Ann's emotional dysfunction. Steven seemed to hold a meaning regarding her behavior that perhaps served as a self-fulfilling prophecy for his emotional needs not being met. Steven's criticism and demands for emotional intimacy perhaps only served to decrease communication and make it harder for Mary Ann to express her emotions.

After a discussion of Mary Ann's family of origin, the therapist ascribed an alternative meaning of "speaking different languages" to Mary Ann's perceived emotional dysfunction. The therapist concluded that the problem may be that Mary Ann speaks a behavioral language, while Steven speaks a verbal language. The conversation ended with the therapist's suggestion that Steven continue speaking in Mary Ann's language by doing things to help, which might continue to encourage Mary Ann's speaking in his language. Mary Ann joined Steven and the therapist, and the original experiment was reassigned.

The couple returned for session three and entered the therapist's office laughing. Each referred to a list of times and events that chronicled their enactment of the suggested experiment. Steven said that he felt closer to Mary Ann, and Mary Ann reported that she was pleased to have Steven involved at home once again. The therapist explored the couple's impressions and promoted the elaboration of how and why the changes were occurring. The therapist, once again, separated the couple, and Mary Ann went first.

SESSION THREE

Excerpt Six

T: I'm really glad things are better. I'm really amazed at the turnaround you two have made.

M: Like I said, it's really great to have Steven back involved with me and the kids again. It feels like a family again. I've been anxious to come here . . . I almost called you. The agree and exaggerate was great.

T: Tell me about it.

M: One time, right after he came home from work, the kids were screaming, the house was a mess, and dinner wasn't even started. Steven said, "I can't believe that you don't have dinner started. You're so disorganized." I said back, "Not only am I disorganized, I can't even control these kids. I'm a terrible mother and wife." Steven looked surprised—and then just simply changed the subject. He didn't say another word about it, he just started helping with dinner.

T: Great. How were you able to resist the temptation to defend yourself and justify the state of things?

M: Well, I just psyched myself up for it, and I was determined to not let him make me upset. But the best one was last Friday night. Steven had a terrifically bad day at work. He lost a major account because of someone else's screwup, and he was very angry. He spent his whole day trying to convince the customer to reconsider, but it didn't work. He was major league bummed out. Well, he came home and was kind of quiet, but I really didn't notice because I was feeding the baby and trying to fix dinner at the same time. Just as we were sitting down to eat, he jumps down my throat and tells me how insensitive I am for not picking up how upset he was. It really bothered me, but I calmed myself, and when he was done I said, "You're right, I am like Mr. Spock and I'll probably always be that way. I guess I wonder how long you're going to put up with me." [Both the therapist and Mary Ann laugh.] As I said it, I got up from the table and walked away to get something from the counter. Steven got up and came over and put his arms around me and reminded me that things were getting better and that he was probably overreacting and should have brought it up himself that he was having a bad day.

T: Wonderful!

M: I was delighted. It was great not to feel crummy about his criticisms. Friday evening turned out great after that. We decided to get a baby-sitter and went out to the movies. [Mary Ann goes out and Steven joins the therapist.]

T: Recall last time in our discussion that you indicated that you would like to find some verbal common ground. I've been thinking about a way for you two to find some common ground, in a verbal way, that is somewhere in between your language and hers. One way may be the marital quid pro quo. It is a communication exercise that promotes honest discussions about the relationship and enables a negotiation of relationship rules. It may be good for you two because it is largely *behavioral* in focus, which may fit better for Mary Ann. It facilitates discussion about the relationship, which is what you've been wanting [Steven nods], but it does so by encouraging a behavioral description of the relationship.

S: Sounds great.

T: Okay, if you're game, let's bounce it off Mary Ann and see what she thinks.

Commentary

The therapist reunited the couple and Steven commented that given their differences in language, he would like to find some common ground on which he and Mary Ann could communicate about their relationship. Mary Ann agreed and said that she was hoping for the same thing. The therapist responded to the couple's request and suggested a communication exercise called "the marital quid pro quo" (Jackson & Lederer, 1968) for the next session.

In session four, the quid pro quo exercise was facilitated by the therapist. The quid pro quo can stimulate a process that is both relationship enhancing and problem solving. It allows a frank discussion of relationship rules, as well as a specific method of negotiation. Briefly, the exercise has four parts: (1) each person says what he or she would like to see more of or less of that would make the marriage more workable, (2) each person repeats the other's list, (3) each person identifies how he or she has negatively contributed to the relationship, and (4) the experience of the exercise itself is discussed.

SESSION FOUR

Excerpt Seven

T: Is there a volunteer to start things up?

S: I'll go first.

T: Steven, please tell your wife what you would like to see more of or less of that would make the marriage more workable for you from your entirely selfish perspective. You have 10 minutes. It's okay to start general and proceed to specific or vice versa. It doesn't matter. Please do not elaborate, explain, or editorialize, just say what you want more of or less of. There will likely be periods of silence for you to collect your thoughts. That's okay. Mary Ann, your job is to listen to your husband and remember what he says, because you will be required to summarize what he says. Please do not say anything. Just maintain comfortable eye contact and listen carefully. Do you both understand? [Both nod]

S: This is hard. I'd like to see more touching, day to day; more hugs; more sharing of feelings; more supportive statements in different things I set out to do; more caring; more able to sense when I'm upset or down, or nervous; less of just not asking about my feelings; more of asking what is bothering me; more of you sharing with me when you're upset about something; more loving words from both of us; more of a desire to be close to me; more initiation on your part to be close to me; more ideas of how to have an intimate evening; more enthusiasm about the relationship; more talking about the future; more discussion of our dreams; less day to day living.

T: Good job. [Therapist repeats instructions to Mary Ann.]

M: I'd like to see more of a family-type relationship; more doing things together for the family; more help around the house and with the kids; more concern for the children; less criticism; more doing things together without the kids; less of the idea that things have to always lead to sex; more doing things without me having to ask you; less of you trying to control my life; doing more things that show me that you love me; more sharing daily life together; more acceptance of me the way I am; more just hanging out together without pressure to talk.

T: Great. [Both Mary Ann and Steven summarize each other's more ofs and less ofs.] Now, Mary Ann, tell your husband all the ways you have contributed in a negative or destructive way to the relationship. You have 5 minutes. It can be past or present things, however you want to fill the time.

M: I have contributed in a negative or destructive way by becoming so involved with taking care of the kids that I neglected you, by being too concerned about everything being "just so." I should have just let things go and tried to pay more attention to you; by withdrawing from you when I was angry, instead of trying harder to talk things out. That's all I can think of.

T: Try and think of one more.

M: I contribute negatively when I let myself get so tired that I shut you and everything else out of my mind.

T: Great. [Therapist repeats instructions to Steven.]

S: I have been destructive to the relationship by putting on too much pressure and making too many demands; by thinking of my own needs and not yours or the kids; by not saying when I'm upset so you know when to try to comfort me; and, finally, by not accepting that we have differences, that you have a different style than I do and I should have tried to work with you instead of against you.

Mary Ann and Steven did very well with the exercise. Mary Ann noted that it was more difficult for her to express her own needs, while Steven noted that it was harder for him to share how he had contributed negatively. Both noted a connection between what they wanted from each other and their own negative contributions; that is, the things they wanted the most were the things that they likely sabotaged by their own behavior. The therapist encouraged further discussion and asked the couple to repeat the exercise and prioritize their lists of "more ofs" and "less ofs."

The therapist planned on negotiating the lists in the next session, but Steven called and cancelled the next appointment. Steven said that Mary Ann and he had agreed that they would like to try things on their own. The therapist was pleased and did not interpret the cancellation in any negative way.

During the phone call with Steven, the therapist commented on the amazing turnaround of the couple and complimented Steven on his hard work. Steven said that he realized that Mary Ann would never live up to his ideal, but that he loved her anyway. The therapist asked permission to follow up to see how they were doing.

On follow-up, Mary Ann reported that everything was still going okay and that, although there had been some rocky times, they seemed better able to deal with the bad times. Mary Ann said that they still used the format of the quid pro quo and that she continued to use the agree and exaggerate strategy. Mary Ann added that not feeling manipulated and controlled allowed her to step back and see how she could initiate more feeling-oriented conversation with Steven.

Discussion

Mary Ann and Steven illustrate the multiple avenues of change that exist in marital therapy. The therapist intervened with both Mary Ann and Steven individually as well as with the couple. The interventions with the couple and Mary Ann were competing experiences, or techniques that seek to alter the context of the actual experience of the problem; clients are asked to do, think, or feel something different. The intervention with Steven involved the therapist's ascription of a different meaning to Mary Ann's difficulties in expressing her feelings. By interviewing separately, the therapist gained access to the idiosyncratic meaning systems of Mary Ann and Steven. Each intervention chosen specifically addressed the client's view of the marital problem, instead of a predetermined theoretical content imposed by the therapist.

The competing experience suggested to the couple (do something without commenting and observe) interrupted the problem-maintaining solution attempts and enabled a context for both to ascribe new meanings to their interactions. The intervention also explicitly validated both their perspectives about the relationship. The couple returned noting several positive occurrences, the most important of which was Steven's expression of hope about the marriage.

The competing experience suggested to Mary Ann (agree and exaggerate) interrupted her ineffective solutions; her behaviorally altered interaction with Steven permitted the ascription of a different meaning. Steven admitted, for the first time, that he could let Mary Ann know when he was feeling down, rather than expecting her to know automatically. The intervention directly validated Mary Ann's perspective of being criticized, and offered her a way to decrease the criticisms in a relationship-enhancing manner.

The therapist-ascribed meaning of "different languages" represented the culmination of a meaning revising conversation with Steven about Mary Ann's emotional dysfunction. The meaning of dysfunction seemed to limit solution alternatives and perpetuate the problem cycle. The therapist offered an alternative meaning in the hopes of permitting a different solution option. The therapeutic dialogue around the meaning of dysfunction led to a different meaning for Mary Ann's communication difficulties, a meaning that resulted in a different solution strategy suggested by Steven (common verbal language of communication). The quid pro quo addressed Steven's request. The alternative meaning validated Steven's view that Mary Ann communicated less verbally than he preferred, and at the same time offered a more benign perspective that led to different remedial action.

9 ❧ Ethical Practice and the Promotion of Change: Maintaining the Balance

RECALL from Chapter 2 that one of the cornerstones of our approach is the strategic model of the MRI (Fisch et al., 1982). The MRI profoundly influenced the field of family therapy by proposing a model free of the encumbrances of a pathology-based perspective, thereby providing an early "wellness" view of the human experience of emotional and interpersonal problems. The significance of that singular contribution can hardly be overstated (Duncan, 1992).

The MRI view, however, has been criticized on ethical grounds for some time and is increasingly under fire in the literature. The interventions of the MRI and other strategic approaches have been argued to be exceedingly instrumental, deceptive, manipulative, and based in a hierarchical position of therapist power and control (cf., Hoffman, 1985; Schwartz, 1989; Slipp, 1989).

As briefly stated in Chapter 5, the limitations inherent in a sole emphasis on strategy has led some to call for a de-focus on intervention and a shift toward the interview process itself. Our response to the criticisms has been to evolve a perspective molded by the ethical challenges of strategic approaches while retaining the aspects that make strategic intervention a viable methodology to the amelioration of human problems.

The multilevel description of change represents an attempt to move beyond the limitations of a sole focus on strategy and expand the intervention process to emphasize in-session meaning revision and the therapeutic relationship. An intention of the multilevel description is to enable a conceptual balance between the promotion of change and ethical clinical practice. While the multilevel description allows a conceptual framework for tempering strategy with relationship considerations, it does not provide pragmatic guidelines for clinical practice.

This chapter presents an overview of the criticisms of a strategic view in several broad areas often identified in the literature: conscious deception, intervention outside of client awareness, paradox, and gender sensitivity. Emerging from a discussion of the clinical application of common factors, a constructivist view, and a meaning system vocabulary of client change, five ethical guidelines are suggested that address the issues of manipulation, power, and paradox. Gender bias is discussed, and suggestions are presented for reducing its impact on the psychotherapy process. Case examples introduced throughout the book are utilized to illustrate the ethical guidelines.

CONSCIOUS DECEIT AND CONSTRUCTIVISM

On the surface, the ethical issue of conscious deceit appears simple and easily summarized: Regardless of theoretical orientation, it is unethical to deceive clients consciously. The previous statement offers little with which to disagree and is further supported by the large body of literature (cited in Chapter 1) regarding the importance of empathy, respect, genuineness, and honesty in the development of a therapeutic relationship (Patterson, 1984). Also, recall that these so-called common factors account for 25%–40% of outcome variance, while technique/orientation variables account for only 15% (Patterson, 1989). Strategic or any other orientation's techniques are largely insignificant next to common factors and client variables. Conscious deceit, therefore, is not only objectionable on a basic moral level, but it also may undermine the core of the therapeutic relationship and interfere with, if not preclude, successful outcome.

It appears, however, that the issue of conscious deceit is not that simple. Despite the fact that strategically oriented authors have condemned deceit for many years, concern continues to be raised, and some therapists may use a strategic orientation to justify deception. Haley (1987) asserts that it is not only naive to believe that one can lie without being caught, but that lying is patronizing and ultimately teaches the client that the therapist is untrustworthy. Clients are often sensitive to incongruities in the therapist's presentation. They may readily perceive the deception contained in an intervention or a therapist that is not genuine. Such a client perception may not only undermine the effectiveness of the intervention, but the therapeutic relationship as well.

Wendorf and Wendorf (1985) suggest that therapists have a variety of choices for being truthful to clients. For example, instead of inventing fictitious treatment teams or team splits when no such disagreements occur, the therapist may honestly present his or her own ambivalence about the client or family's dilemma. O'Hanlon and Wilk (1987) present an exhaustive list of ways they do *not* deceive clients, graphically illustrating a strong position against conscious deception in their work.

Despite these seemingly firm positions, a perception persists that strategic therapy permits one to misrepresent personal beliefs, experiences, and the therapeutic process itself in the service of addressing treatment goals. The existence of this perception has been validated in a study examining ethical dilemmas not addressed by the American Association for Marriage and Family Therapy Code (Green & Hansen, 1989). Some therapists in that study reported that they are willing to manipulate families for therapeutic benefit, even if it meant being dishonest. In another study of therapists' views of paradoxical strategies, Waterson, Gallessich, and Hanson (1987) found a similar pragmatic ethical orientation held by therapists.

Constructivism

This perception may emanate from constructivism and the application of an antirealist epistemology to psychotherapy. Constructivism seems to have been interpreted by some to mean that because truth is a relative phenomenon, and there is no objective reality, misrepresentation (lying) is acceptable when done for benevolent purposes. Given the vulnerability of constructivism to being misinterpreted, a clarification of the contributions of an antirealist epistemology will be discussed that allows for the provision of ethical guidelines.

In Chapter 2, the philosophical position of constructivism and its implications for therapy was discussed. A "common sense" translation was advocated that recognizes the existence of objects, events, and experiences, but challenges hard and fast "objective" understandings about people and problems. Understood in this way, constructivism elevates the client's view of reality, particularly the client's meaning system regarding the presenting problem, to paramount importance in the therapeutic process. The application of constructivism to therapy ascends the client's meaning system to a hierarchically superior position to the therapist's theoretical orientation and/or personal beliefs. Constructivism, therefore, provides a strong rationale for respecting the preeminence of the client's world view. In practical terms, it emphasizes the client's right to be met within his or her idiosyncratic meaning system regarding the reasons that served as the impetus for therapy.

Constructivism should *not* be construed as a rationale for conscious deception or dishonesty. It is the therapist's ultimate responsibility to insure that misrepresentation of the therapist, his or her beliefs, and the therapeutic process does not occur. Because conscious deception is antithetical to respecting the client's meaning system, methods that do not meet the criterion of honest representation should be avoided (Solovey & Duncan, 1992).

Example

Let us return to Joe (from Chapter 3), the 19-year-old student professing to be a messenger from God, for a more in-depth look at the issue of conscious deceit. Recall that the impetus for therapy arose from Joe's persistent efforts at spreading God's word to his parents and neighbors at all hours. Joe's opening comments in therapy were characterized by an insistence upon knowing whether the therapist believed in God and that Joe was a messenger from Him. By agreeing that Joe was indeed a messenger and professing his personal belief, the therapist was able to discuss alternative methods of spreading God's word that were more acceptable to Joe's parents and neighbors.

The therapist did not consciously deceive the client; the therapist responded from a genuine belief in a power higher than humanity and from an abstract view that all people, in one way or another, are called on to be God's messengers or representatives. For the sake of rapport (those disbelieving Joe's messenger status were the devil's disciples), Joe's belief in a unique purpose above and beyond all others was not directly challenged, nor did the therapist affirm Joe's special purpose. The therapist was able to draw upon a personal belief system that permitted the exploration and ultimate selection of competing experiences that empowered Joe to convey his views without hospitalization.

If the therapist did not believe in God or any type of spiritual presence on earth, the therapist would have been engaging in conscious deceit for effect. We believe that regardless of effectiveness, misrepresentation of personal beliefs is unethical. If the therapist did not believe in God, it would have been the therapist's ethical responsibility to develop another method of intervention. For example, the therapist may have responded to Joe's questions of the therapist's belief in God and Joe's messenger role with the following statement:

"While I'm not religious myself and do not think much about my beliefs about God, I do have a deep respect for religious leaders and for people, like you, who believe in God and are willing to lead a life in accordance with their beliefs. Sometimes, unfortunately, people who believe as strongly as you run the risk of being misinterpreted and going unheard."

Such an alternative response may have facilitated a similar exploration of different ways for Joe to spread God's word.

The case of Joe poses additional ethical questions. From the perspective presented in this book, the therapist must not only represent him- or herself honestly, but must also accept and respectfully work within the expressed meaning system of the client. Joe presents a formidable challenge to the acceptance of a client's meaning system. It is asserted here that regardless of what might be considered by some as a "delusional" process, the client has the right of self-determination and holds a perspective of reality that is no less valid than the therapist's. An unusual meaning system or one with which the therapist personally disagrees offers the greatest challenge to placing the client's meaning system in a hierarchically superior position to that of the therapist.

Clients usually do not confront the therapist's personal belief system or ask directly for an opinion about the believability of their position. When a client does ask a direct question, and the therapist honestly disagrees with the client, the therapist must answer in a way that is congruent with his or her personal beliefs, but without disrespect to the client's perspective. As an illustration, consider the client who asked his therapist whether or not he believed that the FBI was monitoring the client's behavior through television. The therapist responded in a manner that was both therapeutic and honest:

"Frankly, it sounds pretty weird to me, and I have to admit that nothing like that has ever happened to me. However, I am not going to tell you that I absolutely know for sure that it is not happening. So how about we take this matter at face value and accept it as it is until we can uncover evidence which proves it one way or another?"

Constructivism and Therapist-Ascribed Meaning

Another implication of a constructivist view (discussed in Chapter 2) is its impact on the therapist's perception of psychotherapy theory. Just as client problems are embedded in the process of creating a structured, predictable reality, therapists may become stuck by overadhering to specific models of therapy that are not applicable in given situations. A constructivist view permits the therapist to discontinue the search for a single therapeutic truth and instead treat models of therapy as somewhat arbitrary metaphorical representations that assist the therapist with organizing his or her thinking about the client's dilemma. Treating models of therapy as views of reality rather than as undeniable truth enables the consideration of multiple views and their situational applicability. This perspective permits the selective ascription of meaning without a belief in the inherent truth of the selected meaning *across* situations. The therapist, however, should believe in the selected meaning in the specific context it is used. This implication does not afford the freedom to say anything at all to clients and remain ethical (or even credible), nor does it allow a therapist to concoct or impose meaning in a haphazard fashion with no regard to its ramifications.

The freedom to select meaning also brings an accompanying ethical responsibility. First, the selected meaning must satisfy the criterion of honest representation; that is, the therapist must believe that the selected meaning is a *plausible* and *credible* explanation of the client's circumstance. For example, suggesting that a client's depression may be related to an unsatisfactory marriage, a set of irrational beliefs, or childhood experiences is only ethical if the therapist genuinely holds the belief that the selected meaning is a possible explanation for the client dilemma. An honest tentativeness in presentation of the meaning permits the client to understand that the therapist is not absolutely certain of the meaning's applicability, as well as allows the client the freedom to disagree.

The selected meaning must also be congruent with the client's stated meaning system, as well as fit the "facts" of the situation. The therapist should attempt to match the client's beliefs, values, and the emotional context associated with the presenting problem. Ethical responsibility is particularly important with therapist-ascribed meaning because the therapist is intervening from outside the client's frame of reference and is introducing elements foreign to the client's meaning system. The therapist must, therefore, be especially sensitive to the client's right to self-determination and nonacceptance of the ascribed meaning, as well as potential negative ramifications. Regardless of the therapist's belief in the fit of the ascribed meaning, *the therapist should not introduce and insist upon the rightness of elements foreign to the client's meaning system* (Solovey & Duncan, 1992).

Example

Joan, described in Chapter 6, represents some of the complexities involved with introduction of elements foreign to the client's meaning system. Remember that Joan seemed to be literally drinking herself to death and sought treatment to address her drinking problem. Exploration of her meaning system through the therapeutic dialogue revealed intense feelings of hatred toward her mother, a long-held belief that Joan's mother permanently damaged her, and an expressed position that childhood abuse at her mother's hands caused her drinking, as well as an inability to change. The therapist accepted the client's meaning system and intervened to assist Joan to stop drinking (her stated goal) by ascribing a different meaning to her drinking and her inability to change. Joan's inability to stop drinking was described as an unconscious way of demonstrating respect for her mother and not showing her up by surpassing her mother's alcohol problem.

The selected meaning of showing respect satisfied the criterion of honest representation, given that the therapist believed the meaning to be a plausible and credible explanation of Joan's circumstances. Joan had been in therapy sporadically for many years addressing her hatred for her mother, as well as her propensity to exacerbate her medical problems with alcohol abuse. Despite previous therapists' admonitions against the drinking and therapeutic attempts to work through Joan's anger and contempt for her mother, the dangerous drinking persisted. In searching for an effective intervention, the therapist selected a meaning that not only fit the facts, but also was plausible to the therapist and matched the client's stated meaning system.

Because an element foreign to the client's stated meaning was introduced, the therapist was especially sensitive to the possible negative ramifications. The meaning was ascribed after Joan explicated her unqualified contempt for her mother. If, on the other hand, Joan had been tentative about her feelings for her mother or was requesting help to address her hatred for her mother, the same ascribed meaning would have been unethical and ineffective. A negative ramification could have been the blaming of the mother and the potential creation or exacerbation of mother–daughter conflict.

The intended result was to empower Joan to use her anger toward her mother, which was accepted as a given by the therapist to stop drinking, rather than as a justification for continued alcohol abuse. Given that the therapist-ascribed meaning came from a frame of reference outside of the client, the therapist would have been obligated to discard the meaning had the client disagreed or did not believe it fit her particular circumstance. Such was not the case with Joan; while she did not like the ascribed meaning, she did not disagree. The ascribed meaning seemed to enable Joan to confront the limitations of her meaning system regarding her mother. Within that context, she changed her drinking pattern on her own.

INTERVENTION OUTSIDE
OF CLIENT AWARENESS

During the past decade a variety of techniques from strategically oriented therapies have been popularized and subsequently criticized for their covert nature. Techniques such as paradox, confusion, rituals, prescription, and hypnosis have been described both as effective and as interventions that inhibit mutuality in the relationship by virtue of their operation outside of the client's awareness.

A representative technique of intervention outside of client awareness is pacing and leading. The therapist mirrors a number of the client's nonverbal gestures and, after a period of time, initiates a nonverbal gesture that is, in turn, followed by the client. The accompanying explanation of this pacing and leading process is that it facilitates a rapport outside of the client's conscious awareness.

Techniques used without clients' input or discussion and that seem to be "done to" clients instead of "done with" raise two ethical concerns: (1) the use of technique outside of client awareness in which no explicit or discussed relationship exists between the technique and the client's goal of therapy; and (2) the attribution of a cause–effect relationship between therapist actions and client response, and the accompanying implication of covert power and control.

These concerns can readily be applied to almost all therapies. Is it ethical to intervene outside of client awareness? Is covert instrumentality an abuse of therapist power and control? Once again, the questions are complex, and consultation of the literature reveals a broad range of opinions.

On one side are those who justify intervention outside of client awareness on several related grounds. Haley (1987) asserts that all therapists, regardless of orientation, conceal information regarding intervention, contending that consideration of timing and depth of intervention would be precluded if therapists revealed all of their ongoing thoughts. While ostensibly proposing full disclosure, therapists carry out unmentioned maneuvers that are concealed from the client (Haley, 1987). Haley also suggests that intervention outside of client awareness is not only appropriate, but is also *more* courteous and respectful than an approach that purports to promote awareness via a therapist sharing his or her interpretation of the client's circumstance. He calls intervention outside of client awareness "courtesy therapy" because it does not force clients to concede to the therapist's formulation of the problem, but rather addresses issues in an indirect way that clients already fully understand.

In contrast, Hoffman (1985) warns against excessive instrumentality and the hierarchical position of power that planned interventions outside of client awareness impose on the therapeutic context. Hoffman (1985) advocates a move away from the highly instrumental position of covertly directive strategic approaches and suggests a cooperative relationship with clients.

This brief sample of the literature provides a snapshot of a recursive dilemma: In one corner is the view that intervention outside of client awareness is not only inevitable, but is also a more ethical position than a perspective that narrows the client's options by imposing the therapist's ideology; in the other corner is the view that such interventions are covertly manipulative, reinforce a therapist position of power, and inhibit collaboration.

Exploration of the dilemma reveals that both sides of the argument have merit. It is impractical, if not ludicrous, to suggest that therapists share all of their ongoing uncensored thoughts with clients. Yet, it is imperative that some boundaries are identified to provide direction for therapists struggling with the ethics of intervention outside of client awareness and covert instrumentality.

Meaning Systems and Interventions
Outside of Client Awareness

Consider the therapeutic process from a meaning systems perspective: The language of meaning and the primacy of the therapeutic alliance guide the therapist through the process of unfolding the client's story and creating a collaborative context for the cogeneration of new meaning. Exploration of the problem and its meaning to the client requires a candid exchange between the therapist and client, as well as a collaborative formulation of outcome criteria that are specified by the client. The therapist may offer a number of ideas for discussion that grow into relevant dialogue or fade away as it becomes apparent that it is not meaningful for the client to pursue; the client's response to therapist-introduced ideas is the indicator of relevance.

In general, the goal is to promote conditions that increase choice and enhance possibilities for revision of those meanings or experiences that the *client* views as problematic. Collaboration from this standpoint is dependent upon the client's *agreement* with what problems will be worked on and criteria for successful problem resolution.

Once the therapist and client agree regarding the criteria for successful therapy, that is, the client's perception of acceptable change concerning the presenting problem, the therapist may suggest an experience or set of experiences that compete with the client's current experience of the problem. Such suggestions promote the construction of different meanings and enable clients to confront the limitations of their meaning systems, thereby facilitating consideration of alternative interpretations of themselves or the problem. Competing experiences merely provide the opportunity for revision to occur and, therefore, rely on the inherent resources of the client and human tendency to attribute meaning to experience.

Direct exploration of the client's experience of the presenting problem may also promote an alternative ascription of meaning *by the client*. Clients sometimes generate new meanings and make new distinctions and connections as the therapeutic conversation unfolds, and, therefore, no competing experience or therapist-ascribed meanings are suggested. Such client-ascribed meanings that lead to problem resolution are viewed as the best possible treatment outcome because of minimal therapist involvement.

The language of meaning systems enables a nonpurposive and noninterfering language for change, as well as suggests some ethical direction regarding intervention outside of client awareness. The therapist's role is collaborative and involves the promotion of conditions that make a revision of meaning possible. New meaning is not dictated or instrumentality forced; the client is always perceived as having freedom of choice, and the therapist works to expand rather than limit client choices. The client's input is essential and therefore solicited throughout any intervention sequence.

When the client benefits from a therapist's suggestion of a competing experience, it is clearly the client who has idiosyncratically constructed the new meaning and performed the work necessary for change to occur. The therapist is instrumental only in the sense that a deliberate attempt is made to set a context for change and empower clients to challenge their meaning systems in the hope that alternatives will be discovered independently.

Therapist intervention, therefore, is not considered instrumental in a cause–effect way with the observed change. Rather, the observed change is seen only in the purview of the client and the client's interactional experience of doing, feeling, and/or thinking something different in regard to the presenting problem. Consequently, collegial discussion of client change must necessarily include interactional descriptions of the change and attribute credit to the client. Therapy only provides opportunity for change.

While the therapist is candid in the mutual discussion of meanings and experiences the client desires to change, the therapist does not comment on the theory of meaning construction or other theoretical contents underlying intervention. Concealment is not grounded in the belief that clients should not be informed on this level of abstraction, but rather because: (1) the therapist's philosophical/theoretical position is not relevant and may shift the therapeutic conversation away from the client; and (2) disclosure of such information reinforces the "expert" role of the therapist and may be viewed as disrespectful by the client, interfering with the collaborative exploration required for intervention (Solovey & Duncan, 1992).

The language of meaning systems also provides guidance regarding intervention outside of client awareness. Through the therapeutic conversation, clients make explicit their thoughts, feelings, and actions regarding the problem(s) that brought them to therapy. Most often, clients articulate the meanings related to changing the presenting problem and how they may experience such changes. While the therapist may not disclose his or her own interpretation of how an intervention may be helpful, the therapist intervenes only with meanings and experiences that are mutually agreed upon and generally relies on the client's judgment regarding experiences that are relevant for discussion and intervention. This does not preclude the therapist holding alternative views of the client's circumstances nor necessitate introduction of these alternatives to the therapeutic process. Rather, it only requires the therapist to apply those alternative views to the client's explicated goal for therapy. Movement beyond the client's agreed-upon initial goals must be through a continual process of negotiation.

It is our position that *the therapist should intervene only with outcome criteria that are mutually agreed upon by the therapist and client*, and there needs to be an explicit relationship in the therapist's mind between the intervention (ascribed meaning or competing experience) chosen and the client's articulation of the presenting problem. While operation outside of client awareness is necessary to a degree, intervention in an area not discerned to be a problem by the client is disrespectful. For example, intervention in a client's marriage when it has not been discussed by the client as relevant to the presenting problem constitutes an attempt to influence without client permission, and should therefore be avoided. From the position presented here, the therapist only has license to attempt influence in meanings and experiences that have been mutually explored and agreed to be relevant to the problem that brought the client to therapy.

Just as conscious deceit negatively affects outcome by undermining common factors, intervention on goals not agreed upon by the client is similarly counterproductive to successful outcome. As stated in Chapter 3, there is a large body of evidence that the therapeutic alliance, as rated from client, therapist, and third-party perspectives, is the *best* predictor of outcome (Alexander & Luborsky, 1986). Recall that the therapeutic alliance consists of relationship factors and is a function of the degree of agreement between the therapist and client *about the goals and tasks* of psychotherapy (Bordin, 1979). The therapist imposition of goals may, therefore, be counterproductive to successful outcome.

Example

Remember Richard, who suspected his wife of having an affair after discovering footprints in the snow. Other bits of evidence led Richard to check the bedsheets for signs of semen. After finding a stain, Richard went to a laboratory, where tests confirmed his suspicions. Throughout the process, Richard's wife denied having an affair and argued that the semen was Richard's. Her rebuttal contained counteraccusations that Richard was paranoid and sick. Richard's distress led him to miss work, and he was eventually placed on sick leave and referred for therapy by the company doctor.

In response to Richard's presenting problem, the therapist accepted and validated the client's meaning system. This permitted Richard to calm down and establish the goal of returning to work. This rapid shift occurred after the therapist ascribed the meaning of "inadvertently proving his wife right" to the variety of things that Richard was doing that confirmed his wife's declaration of his craziness, namely, not working, obtrusively checking on her, trying to convince everyone he wasn't crazy, etc. Disconfirming accusations of craziness entailed returning to work, backing off of his accusations, spending positive time with his kids, and waiting patiently for the results of the DNA test.

The therapist-ascribed meaning in this case was not conscious deception; the therapist believed that there was validity to Richard's story. The selected meaning of proving his wife right satisfied the criterion of honest representation, given that the therapist believed the meaning to be a plausible and credible explanation of Richard's circumstances. Despite the company doctor's admonitions against his suspicions, Richard continued his mistrust and self-destructive path. In searching for an effective intervention, the therapist selected a meaning that not only fit the facts, but also was plausible to the therapist and matched the client's stated meaning system.

Because an element foreign to the client's stated meaning system was introduced, the therapist was especially sensitive to the possible negative ramifications. The meaning was ascribed after Richard explicated his unqualified mistrust for his wife. If, on the other hand, Richard had been tentative about his feelings for his wife or was requesting marital therapy, the same ascribed meaning would not have been appropriate. A negative ramification could have been the blaming of the wife and the potential creation or exacerbation of conflict.

The intended result of the ascribed meaning (proving his wife right) and the competing experience (behavioral suggestions) was to empower Richard to use his mistrust of his wife to care for himself and return to work rather than as a justification for the continued self-defeating behaviors of constant surveillance and missing work. Given that the ascribed meaning came from a frame of reference external to the client, the therapist would have been obligated to discard the meaning had Richard not accepted it or did not believe it fit his circumstances.

Such was not the case for Richard. Richard returned to work and spent positive time with his kids. He monitored his wife's behavior but did not confront her. Richard ultimately dropped the DNA test, accepting that he knew in his heart that his wife had an affair. He concluded that he wanted out of the marriage and filed for divorce.

The ascribed meaning and competing experience set the conditions

for Richard's behaviorally altered interaction within his social environment. He confronted the limitations of his course of action and reached
his own conclusions about his marriage independent of the therapist.

The therapist's behavior was instrumental in the sense that he
enabled the context for change by providing the therapeutic alliance
(common factors and agreement of goals and tasks) and by promoting the
conditions for change (ascribed meaning and competing experience).
The client independently did the work required for problem improvement.

The competing experience in the form of behavioral suggestions was
not prescribed so that the client would resist or do the opposite. Even the
therapist's suggestion of continuing the DNA test was not intended to
promote a reverse psychology response from Richard. From a meaning
system perspective, the therapist wanted the client to follow the
suggestions to set up a context for revisions in the client's meaning system
regarding his actions about his wife's affair. Enlisting cooperation and
input from the client and attempting to create the conditions for change
represent an antithetical point of view to power, resistance, and
adversarial views of so-called paradoxical interventions. Not only are
resistance or power explanations of paradox as a "thing" that is done to
clients ethically suspect, such explanations are also problematic from a
conceptual point of view.

Paradox: Actual or Attributed

Paradox has been defined as a contradiction that follows correct
deductions from consistent premises (Watzlawick, Beavin, & Jackson,
1967). Consider the following statement, which is sometimes termed a
true paradox. The statement, "This sentence is false," is a true paradox
because of its contradictory and self-reflexive comment on itself. This
self-reflexive loop is troublesome because it essentially denies itself,
thereby creating havoc with the ability to organize and gain control over
the information presented through language. It is, therefore, said to
constitute a paradox.

During recent years, some theorists have suggested that there is an
alternative explanation for paradox. Rather than an entity in and of itself,
paradox may be a description by an observer of an apparently
contradictory phenomenon (Cronen, Johnson, & Lannamann, 1982;
Dell, 1981). Paradox then exists only in the concepts of the observer and
is not an innate property of the action. Dell (1981) argues, "By definition,
paradox must always be tied to an observer for whom the situation or
question is 'paradoxical' " (p. 127). In other words, the phenomenon of
paradox requires the beliefs, values, opinions, expectations, and common
sense of the observer. Consequently, paradox, like beauty, lies solely in

the eyes of the beholder and is entirely relative to the world view of the observer. Action deemed paradoxical by an observer may not seem so to those involved in the event under observation.

Reconsider the statement, "This sentence is false." As discussed previously, this statement can be argued to represent a true paradox. Cronen et al. (1982), however, have demonstrated the relativity of paradox by describing the Taoist perspective on that statement. They describe the Eastern philosophical view that language is inherently obstructive of enlightenment and quote Lao-Tse's dictum, "He who speaks knows not; he who knows, speaks not." From the Taoist view, then, the statement, "This sentence is false," presents an innate and fundamental truth that is consistent with all Taoist philosophical premises (Cronin et al., 1982).

Example

Recall Janice (introduced in Chapter 5) who entered therapy because of her fear of flying. To address Janice's stated goal of reducing her fears and feeling in control, the therapist suggested that Janice spend 15–30 minutes considering the dangers of flying and feeling her fears intensely. Some therapists may describe such a symptom prescription as indeed paradoxical because the therapist is asking the client to engage in the very problem that the client is attempting to resolve. It looks like a paradox because it appears contradictory to therapeutic goals and defies what some orientations may consider logical action. Some may describe the intervention with Janice as a way of double binding her, paradoxing her, or in other words, attempting to influence Janice to do the opposite of what the therapist is suggesting. Such "paradoxing" is usually justified in the literature with clients whose resistance is high and motivation is low (e.g., Stanton, 1981). In our view, if resistance is high and motivation is low, then it is likely more related to therapeutic neglect of the relationship, the choice of intervention, and the therapist's style of presentation rather than some quality attributable to the client.

No paradox was observed by the therapist who suggested the prescription with Janice. The suggestion was based upon a consistent theory, a set of guiding assumptions, and from information obtained from Janice that her primary solution attempt was avoiding her fears altogether. Based upon a process-constructive, relationship-oriented frame of reference, the prescription was offered in the hope that it would create a contextual competition that would allow Janice to reach alternative meanings or solutions regarding her fear of flying.

Even if Janice had followed the suggestion and not experienced the hoped-for revision, it would have demonstrated to her that she could exercise some control over her fears, given that she deliberately made them happen and was able to face them directly. If Janice chose not to follow the assignment, then no harm would have occurred. The therapist would have been open to client input, explored its meaning, and pursued another path to meaning revision. Because of the therapist's beliefs and expectations, the prescription did not seem paradoxical, because no contradiction of a prevailing methodology occurred (Fraser, 1984b).

Janice also did not view the therapist's suggestion as contradictory to her goals and indicated to the therapist her agreement with the prescription. The suggestion seemed to allow Janice to experience her fears without trivializing or invalidating them, which opened the door for Janice to not only view her flying fears as valid, but also to share her concerns with others for the first time.

Just as the therapist must proceed cautiously when introducing elements that are foreign to the client's meaning system, equal care should be taken when suggesting competing meaning experiences. In this sense, the frame of reference that the therapist uses to organize his or her thinking about an assignment and the therapist's expectations related to follow-through are of paramount importance. Although a revision in meaning may occur whether or not the client decides to enact the suggestion, *the therapist should not make a suggestion and expect that the client will not enact it* (Solovey & Duncan, 1992). Doing so undermines the collaborative nature of the therapeutic alliance, implies covert power, and in some circumstances could lead to harm, if the client surprised the therapist and carried through on a suggestion that was not supposed to be followed. Competing experiences should be designed as no-lose situations for the client.

ETHICAL GUIDELINES: CONSCIOUS DECEIT AND INTERVENTIONS OUTSIDE OF CLIENT AWARENESS

From the examination of constructivism and a meaning system perspective, five ethical guidelines emerge regarding conscious deceit, interventions outside of client awareness, and paradox:

1. Therapists should not consciously deceive clients.
2. Therapists should not introduce and insist upon the rightness of elements foreign to the client's meaning system.
3. Therapists should not place undue emphasis on therapist power and control by assigning a cause–effect relationship to therapist intervention and client change.
4. Therapists should not intervene outside of client awareness on meanings or experiences that are not mutually agreed upon by the therapist and client.

5. Therapists should not make a suggestion and expect that the client will not enact it.

Limitations

Throughout this book we have emphasized the limitations inherent in any single theoretical orientation of psychotherapy. Elevation of the client's meaning system to a superior position to the therapist's theoretical frame of reference makes possible a selective integration of theories and techniques that best fit the client. But here too, the therapist must be wary of contradictions that may arise from an overly rigid adherence to an invariant elevation of client meaning systems.

There are several somewhat extreme, but obvious, situations that preclude elevating the client's meaning system and not insisting upon the validity of the therapist's point of view. Examples include sexual abuse, any act of violence, or involuntary hospitalization. In these instances, the therapist must necessarily insist upon the rightness of safety and nonviolence. These types of cases warrant special consideration and several ethical concerns must be weighed (e.g., client welfare, therapist trustworthiness, client autonomy, protection of society, etc.). It is beyond the scope of this chapter to address these special cases, and the reader is referred to other publications (Beauchamp & Childress, 1983; Bok, 1978).

While certain cases warrant special concern, they do not necessarily negate placing the client's meaning system in higher regard than the therapist's personal beliefs or theoretical orientation. For example, a client professing to be a messenger from God, sent to avenge Him by killing sinners, will likely require the therapist to act as an agent of social control. On the other hand, a client such as Joe, professing to be a messenger from God, sent to spread God's love may not require any act of social control by the therapist.

GENDER BIAS AND PSYCHOTHERAPY

The MRI model has also been recently criticized on the basis of gender insensitivity. Walsh and Scheinkman (1989) assert:

> The MRI brief therapy model has been developed exclusively by men and . . . appeals more to male than female therapists. The MRI model was . . . adorned with rational, abstract, impersonal language and metaphors. Also, the model's instrumental nature and narrow focus, as well as its emphasis on behavior and cognition, omit important aspects of women's connected ways of learning and knowing, which utilize contextual understanding, interpretation, and self-knowledge. (p. 17)

These criticisms are reflective of a larger concern that not only are approaches to psychotherapy insensitive to gender difference, but more important, are theoretically and pragmatically reinforcing the status quo of gender oppression (Hare-Mustin, 1987). Men's roles have been historically associated with greater power and privilege, as well as greater social value. The problem arises in the application of these social, political, historical, and psychological phenomena to clinical practice. Identification of the problem of gender oppression unfortunately does not provide definitive explanations regarding how to address best the problem in psychotherapy. Despite a therapist's best intentions, gender bias may be introduced to the therapy process.

The struggle to maintain a balance between promoting change and ethical practice is further complicated by the problem of gender bias. On one hand, an approach that ignores the role of differential power in problem generation and resolution is woefully inadequate. For example, minimizing the financial constraints on some women attempting to leave relationships is readily condemnable. On the other hand, an approach that invariably addresses gender oppression across cases seems to obscure the diversity of women's lives; an emphasis on gender roles as necessarily constricting opportunities and blocking self-expression ignores the possibility that not all individuals find prescribed roles oppressive or confining (Hare-Mustin & Maracek, 1990).

Gender bias is indeed another challenge that a therapist must routinely face. Assistance with the gender challenge has been recently provided by Hare-Mustin and Maracek's (1990) provocative discussion of gender theory viewed through a constructivist lens. They assert that, like all others, gender theories are but representations of reality that organize particular assumptive frameworks and reflect certain interests; ideas about gender differences are social constructions. Hare-Mustin and Maracek argue that conventional meanings ascribed to gender have tended to focus on difference and that such a focus is inherently biased and limited.

Hare-Mustin and Maracek propose two biases in gender theory that not only help understanding of the complexities involved in applying gender theory to clinical practice, but also provide some guidance in that application. The following discussion presents the contrasting gender biases, namely, alpha and beta biases, and provides our interpretation and application to clinical practice illustrated by a case example from this book.

Alpha Bias

Alpha bias is defined as the tendency to exaggerate differences between men and women (Hare-Mustin & Maracek, 1990). Exaggeration occurs when gender differences are emphasized, while similarities are excluded. Alpha bias permits the recognition of women's unique capacities for relationships and the richness of women's inner experience. Alpha bias has the positive effect of countering the cultural devaluation of women and encouraging greater self-acceptance (Hare-Mustin & Maracek, 1990).

Yet, emphasis on difference to the exclusion of similarity is fraught with two related pitfalls. An emphasis on difference can lead to a logic that inadvertently supports stereotypes that have been used to exploit women; a focus on difference can support the status quo by denying that change is needed in the structure of work and family life (Gilder, 1987). For example, consider the traditional view that women are better suited for caretaking roles. Such a presumed view of gender difference masks the inequality between men and women and the disparate power that exists between caretaking and breadwinning roles. Difference can be used to justify unequal treatment of males and females and, therefore, perpetuate stereotypical and restrictive roles. The possibility that it is the unequal treatment that may lead to the apparent difference is consequently hidden from view (Hare-Mustin & Maracek, 1990). Probably at its worst logical extreme, the emphasis on difference can foster solidarity among men, and the overall culture, in the view that women are a deviant "out group" (Beauvoir, 1953). Exaggerated differences can open the way for discounting women's legitimate concerns and/or pathologizing the presumed differences. For example, consider the emotional lability that accompanies premenstrual syndrome (PMS) in some women. While a diagnosis of PMS can provide a helpful understanding of emotional lability, and in some women, can lead to helpful treatment, PMS can also be open to the negative consequences of alpha bias. Through the understanding that PMS results in emotional outbursts solely related to hormonal changes, the stage is set for men to discount and invalidate the legitimate distress and concerns of women attempting to express themselves. Women, therefore, are treated as if their concerns have no validity because of the PMS; the status quo is maintained, and the situation is primed for an escalating and painful cycle of disqualified attempts to be heard.

Consider the gender difference that women demonstrate more caring and concern for relationships, often assuming the majority of responsibility for their well-being. In reiteration, such a presumed gender difference obscures unequal treatment and the disparate power associated with men's and women's roles. The observed difference may be better explained by an individual's relative position in the social hierarchy (Wilden, 1972); that is, taking care of a relationship seems quite reasonable from a position of no power and no other apparent choices. In addition, exaggerating the difference can lead to the ascription of pathology to the perceived difference. Caring, concern, and responsibility for a relationship, when highlighted in particular ways, can become co-dependency, overinvolved mother, or other labels that transform presumed gender differences into gender deficits.

Another pitfall associated with alpha bias is that it leads to the minimization of the differences or variability *among* women. Viewing women as a set of so-called feminine traits ignores the complexity and diversity of an individual woman's experience. Men are usually viewed as individuals, while women are generally seen as women and largely homogeneous (Park & Rothbart, 1982). Just as diagnostic labels may provide useful generalities while not capturing the essence and beauty of variation, reducing the richness of women to gender differences is similarly nondescriptive and restrictive.

Beta Bias

Just as alpha bias has positive utility and negative consequences, beta bias, the minimization of differences, similarly has both helped and hindered the oppression of women. On the positive side, minimizing differences and gaining equal treatment under the law has enabled women to gain greater access to educational and occupational opportunities. The argument for no difference, however, carries an accompanying conse-quence of drawing attention away from women's special needs and the difference in power and resources between men and women (Hare-Mustin & Maracek, 1990). Ignoring differences has historically resulted in theories of development, psychology, and psychiatric diagnoses that base norms of human behavior solely on male experience, or in theories that assign equal responsibility, influence, and power to situations in which women tend to hold less power and have fewer choices.

For example, consider the extent to which rationality, logic, unemotionality, and control/modulation of emotions (traditionally male characteristics) are significant to psychiatric diagnosis and also how women tend to comprise the majority of certain diagnoses. Recall Anita's emotional expressive style and her hospitalization and subsequent diagnosis of borderline personality disorder. The hospital therapist suggested that Anita's husband stay calm when Anita expressed her anger or was out of control. This directive may be construed as the imposition of the male norm that calm and rational is healthy, while the expression of emotion is not. Anita was, unfortunately, set up by this traditional and narrow view of healthy functioning to find herself in an endless cycle of invalidation of not only her concerns about her marriage, but also her way of being and relating. Ignoring difference and using male-based norms is inherently an inequitable state of affairs.

System theories have also been subject to beta bias. System theorists have attempted to dismiss the concept of differential power, asserting that both individuals in a relationship contribute to the maintenance of that relationship. The notion of reciprocity implies that the individuals are not only involved, but equally involved in maintaining interaction and equally influencing its outcome. Such a view obscures the social and economic conditions that contribute to the unequal distribution of power and resources between men and women, and how such conditions tend to restrict women's options (MacKinnon & Miller, 1987). For example, consider the woman that does not work outside of the home who is involved in a battering relationship. A view that such a woman is equally capable of leaving the relationship as the wage-earning batterer, or that the woman has equal influence over stopping the battering cycle is incomprehensible.

A final example of how ignoring differences or treating men and women equally is not always equitable is provided by no fault divorce settlements. While presumably providing equal (no difference) treatment under the law, such settlements were found to raise men's standard of living by 42%, while lowering women and children's by 73% (Weitzman, 1985). Beta bias, to paraphrase Orwell, demonstrates that while men and women are equal, men are sometimes more equal than women.

Preventing Alpha and Beta Biases

The challenge of preventing gender bias begins with the recognition that constructing gender differences with clients has both positive and negative implications. While ostensibly helping women, highlighting the uniqueness of women and minimizing the difference between men and women both can contribute to maintenance of the status quo of oppression. Gender viewed as a dichotomy discounts the complexity of human action and shields both men and women from the disconcerting recognition of inequality (Hare-Mustin & Maracek, 1990).

Gender theory (actually a set of several theories), while providing an invaluable counterpart to traditional male-dominated positions, has been largely a theory of difference. Like all other theories of human behavior, it is inherently limited and posits no special truth that stretches across the range and diversity of clients that clinicians routinely encounter. Gender theory, then, requires discriminant application just as does psychoanalytic, behavioral, or other specific theories. Therapist reformulation of the client's informal theory regarding the presenting concern into formal gender theory and pursuing an invariant path will lead to the same predictable results as will sole reliance on any perspective: Some clients will get better, some will drop out or get worse, and some will stay the same. Viewing gender theory as a theory of difference, or one explanation among many possibilities to be explored selectively with clients, constitutes a first step toward preventing gender bias.

Gender bias can be avoided by the therapist's adoption of a cautious and respectful stance regarding perceived differences that emerge in the therapeutic conversation. The client description may be conceptualized as a gender difference, but also in terms of the client's differential access to power and resources, position in the social hierarchy, or other explanation unrelated to any formal theory. Avoiding alpha bias requires the therapist to be open to multiple explanations and meanings without being wedded to any one specific meaning.

When gender difference seems relevant to the evolving dialogue between the therapist and client, the therapist may ascribe such a meaning for the client's consideration. The ascription of gender difference may lead to a cogeneration of new meanings, or it may fade away as irrelevant if the client indicates by his or her response that it is not meaningful to pursue. Just as any other situation in which an element novel to the meaning system of the client is ascribed, it is unethical to introduce gender difference and insist upon its inherent rightness. The client is the ultimate judge of what is right. Gender sensitivity is critical to the therapeutic process; placing gender theory above the client's meaning system regarding the presenting problem is antithetical to our view of empathy and respect.

Alpha bias can also be prevented by the therapist's reluctance to label or categorize so-called gender traits in such a way that they become gender deficits. Recognition that some labels seem to be caricatures of feminine traits that pathologize presumed differences can help the therapist to remain cautious in using such labels. This does not mean, however, that such labels may not be useful or helpful to discuss at times with some clients, especially with clients who introduce the label for discussion or who already identify with the label.

Finally, alpha bias may be avoided through the appreciation of the uniqueness of the individual, the beauty of human variation, and the inherent power, wisdom, and strength that clients possess. Alpha bias is prevented by reliance on the client's judgment regarding what topics are relevant to the presenting problem, including whether or not the client feels oppressed or restricted by gender roles. Just as in other situations in which the therapist may hold a different, or several different views of the client's problem, it is unethical to intervene in areas not identified as a problem by the client. The therapist has license only to attempt influence in presumed gender differences if those differences have been mutually explored and agreed to be relevant to the problem that served as the impetus for therapy.

Beta Bias

Preventing beta bias is probably the more difficult because it is somewhat confusing to understand how treating men and women equally can result in gross inequities when examined at a different level. In many ways, prescriptive equality is an ideal that is rarely applicable to the harsh socioeconomic conditions within which women and certain minorities are embedded. Equality may be legislated and personally strived for by the individual therapist in his or her work, but the larger cultural context often dictates less-than-equal conditions for those who are not white males; a middle socioeconomic status (SES) white boy will enjoy a myriad of opened doors and will have access to resources that are simply nonexistent for a lower SES minority girl. Consequently, these larger contexts must be recognized by the therapist and considered as part of any perspective that advocates for or presumes equality. Believing that men and women are equal on one level must be tempered with the more-than-likely possibility that they are not equal on another level. For example, advocating that abused women leave abusive relationships without recognition and exploration of what they will face thereafter does little more than satisfy the therapist's fantasy of the way things should be.

Conclusions

Remaining gender sensitive and open to the unfolding of gender meaning while not introducing alpha and beta biases offers yet another tightrope on which a therapist must walk. Placing the client's meaning system in a superior position to the therapist's personal values and theoretical orientation goes a long way toward remaining sensitive to gender, while avoiding gender bias. Allowing the client to select the goals and direct the conversational content reduces the risk of therapist-imposed gender biases.

Expanding the model of the MRI to include both meaning revision and relationship aspects increases sensitivity to gender by addressing some women's unique capacities for relationships and connected ways of learning; the multilevel description of change is inclusive of the more intuitive components of the change process. The language of meaning systems promotes and empowers client self-knowledge and interpretation, and fosters a more egalitarian therapist–client relationship, given the therapist's utter dependence on the client's input to the process and total reliance on the client's resources and strengths. The desire for a collaborative person-to-person relationship does not discount the differential power inherent in therapist–client context, but rather attempts to utilize therapist power to provide the conditions that enable clients to make satisfactory lives for themselves, rather than to promote a particular way for clients to live.

Hare-Mustin and Maracek (1990) end their stimulating discussion with a provocative conclusion:

> We end by recalling that theories persist as they are useful . . . gender difference is no longer useful . . . We look to a paradigm shift that transcends dualisms of mind and nature, freedom and determinism, individual and society, men and women. By recognizing that experience, purpose, and meaning are embedded in ongoing social relations. . . . The description of old categories and practices opens the way for new interpretations and meanings. (pp. 198–199)

In many ways, we believe that transcending the dualism of gender can be accomplished by entering into a relationship with the individual as an individual first—and then contemplating the relevancy of gender guided by the needs of that individual and the meanings that unfold and evolve via the validating context of therapeutic conversation.

Example

Recall Mary from Chapter 5 and her desire to return her husband to his previous way of behaving. Her husband had recently begun coming home late and going out more frequently at night. Mary wondered whether or not her husband was having an affair and began holding a vigil each night waiting for her husband to arrive home.

Gender difference was one of several ways the therapist conceptualized Mary's situation, given that in many ways Mary's marriage could be described as a traditional male-dominated relationship with sharp demarcation of roles and the differential power that accompanies breadwinning versus caretaking roles. The therapist did not comment on the hypothesized gender difference, but rather filed it for future consideration. By allowing Mary to unfold her narrative, it became clear that she did not see her role as confining or restrictive or herself as a victim of oppression in any way. All of Mary's comments regarding herself and her family life were reflective of satisfaction except for her husband's recent patterns and her fear of an affair.

As therapy progressed, it also became clear that her sole objective was to return things to their previous state; Mary was worried about her marriage and would do anything to save it. Respecting that goal and validating her "save the marriage" mission helped the therapist prevent alpha bias and focused the therapist's suggestions toward Mary's reason for being in therapy. The therapist did not label Mary's behavior as co-dependent or use any other label that implies blame or exaggerates presumed gender differences. As the process progressed, the therapist learned of Mary's friend suggesting that Mary must be co-dependent to continue in the relationship with her husband. Mary took great offense at this statement, and, had the therapist introduced that label before allowing Mary's views to be expressed, it may have undermined the therapeutic relationship.

By focusing on, accepting, and validating Mary's meaning system— essentially taking that meaning system as the frame of reference for therapy—the therapist was able to offer a suggestion that assisted Mary to achieve her purpose. Through that validation process and Mary's behaviorally altered interaction with her husband, Mary was able to empower herself to reorganize her meaning system about herself and her relationship. Mary became active in relationships and activities outside of her marriage and decided to pursue her own growth. She accomplished these changes independent of her husband, her therapist, and without the therapist introducing gender difference.

SUMMARY

This chapter has attempted to provide some ethical direction in the broad areas of conscious deceit, intervention outside of client awareness, paradox, and gender sensitivity. Emerging from changes in the field toward a reemphasis on the therapeutic alliance, ethical challenges of strategic therapy in the literature, and our own training and clinical experiences, five ethical guidelines were offered to address the thorny topics of manipulation, power, and control.

By emphasizing a meaning system vocabulary of client change, the internal language of the therapist was linked to an ethical practice of therapy. How the therapist thinks about what he or she is doing with clients and why, makes a subtle yet distinct difference as to the degree of flexibility the therapist may ethically exercise when addressing the meaning systems of clients. Constructivism is a tool that, when used properly, increases therapist flexibility, serves as a rationale for placing the client's meaning system in a hierarchically superior position to the theoretical orientation of the therapist, and allows for a language about change that deemphasizes therapist power and control.

Alpha and beta biases were introduced as contradictions that may impair the therapist's ability to be gender sensitive. Exaggerating or minimizing differences can create a conceptual trap that inadvertently supports gender oppression. Developing an approach that goes beyond these biases requires a general openness to unfolding gender or cultural meanings as they emerge in the therapeutic dialogue. Through this unfolding process, the therapist can become attuned to gender and cultural meanings as they relate to the client's presenting problem. Allowing gender and cultural meanings to fade from the therapeutic conversation when they are not deemed as relevant by the client reduces the potential for an imposition of bias.

10 ⛾ Summary and Conclusions

HIS book represents our struggle to integrate clinical experience and the diversity of theories and techniques into a coherent framework for practice. Clinical experience taught us three conceptually simple, yet pragmatically difficult, lessons: (1) all theoretical models have limited applicability; (2) the therapeutic relationship is more valuable than expert interventions; and (3) what clients think, feel, and want has more relevance than our favored academic conceptualizations. Clients taught us these lessons in humility, which served as the impetus to reassess our work and search for more satisfactory descriptions of clinical practice.

Eclecticism, common factors, and brief therapy emerged as significant influences that not only matched our clinical experience, but also provided direction in the quest for a reliable and flexible intellectual framework to guide therapy with individuals, couples, and families. Eclecticism emphasizes the explanatory and predictive inadequacy of any one theoretical school. Common factors and their outcome effects underscore the importance of the therapeutic relationship and the relative insignificance of specific technique or theoretical content. Finally, brief therapy highlights the values of efficiency and efficacy in clinical practice.

Evolving from the interaction of our clinical experience and the three empirical influences came the process constructive theoretical foundations discussed in Chapter 2. The different perspectives of process (i.e., process level systems, interactive process around the problem, and the process/content distinction) reflect the flexibility of eclecticism, an emphasis on the interpersonal system of the therapeutic relationship, and a focus on the problem presentation itself. All three descriptions comprise a formal theory that allows for maximum incorporation of the idiosyncratic presentation of the client; process descriptions enable a relatively content-free theory for practice. Constructivism reinforces a content-free perspective and provides a rationale for the outright primacy of the client's experience, internal frame of reference, and goals in therapy. Constructivism also supports an eclectic perspective, given that theories of psychotherapy are viewed as no more than metaphorical representations that merit consideration, but not invariant application.

The three sources of influence are central to our theory, pragmatic assumptions, and clinical application. Given their importance, we encouraged the reader to evaluate the approach in this book on dimensions derived from the three sources: (1) Goldfried and Newman's (1986) identified themes as important to eclecticism, (2) operationalization of the common factors of psychotherapy, and (3) adherence with Budman and Gurman's (1988) value ideals of brief therapy. This chapter provides our own evaluation and presents our conclusions regarding the future of psychotherapy.

THEMES OF ECLECTICISM

Given that the presented approach purports to be eclectic, Goldfried and Newman's five themes provide a useful method of evaluation. The themes are (1) the potential complementarity of the divergent approaches to therapy; (2) the interactional significance of cognition, behavior, and affect; (3) the need for a common theoretical language; (4) the elucidation of universal meta-theoretical principles of human change; and (5) a desire for an empirically based procedure.

Complementarity of Divergent Approaches

This theme is best summarized by Pinsof's (1983) assertion that "each modality and orientation has its particular 'domain of expertise,' and that these domains can be interrelated to maximize their assets and minimize their deficits" (p. 20).

The theme of complementarity is present in several schemes for integrating differing orientations and methods (e.g., Driscoll, 1984; Pinsof, 1983; Wachtel, 1977), including our earlier strategic behavioral integration, in which the MRI compliance-enhancing strategies complemented the behavioral domain of skill acquisition (Duncan et al., 1987). While these schemes enhance flexibility and broaden therapeutic options, they are inherently restricted by the formal theory or theoretical content from which they are constructed.

Complementarity among approaches may be further enhanced by a reliance on the client's vantage point that is unencumbered by a search for theoretical compatibility. Conceptualizing complementarity from the client's perspective enables all models of psychotherapy to be potentially complementary.

Recall Ted from Chapter 6, whose desire to understand his anxiety and the available treatment options was addressed by the therapist presentation of psychoanalytic, behavioral, existential, and family systems perspectives. Ted considered the applicability of the different views in the context of a symptom prescription and idiosyncratically concluded that the anxiety was related to the boredom of his job and the lack of romance in his marriage. Ted essentially combined the existential and family systems perspectives in a unique way that would have never occurred to the therapist. Although one may speculate that the two approaches are theoretically complementary at some level, the question of formal theory complementarity is largely irrelevant. Complementarity, as in the case of Ted, is best determined by the client's response and judgment. Ted essentially formulated a new theory with explanatory and predictive validity for his specific circumstance.

Interaction of Cognition, Behavior, and Affect

This theme is reflective of attempts to move beyond an invariant emphasis on cognition, behavior, or affect, to an approach that: (1) emphasizes the *interaction* of cognitions, behavior, and affect (e.g., Schwartz, 1982); and (2) concentrates on one component over another as a function of client characteristics instead of the therapist's orientation (e.g., Driscoll, 1984). Goldfried and Newman (1986) point toward a three-dimensional schema that recognizes the "complex interdependence of thinking, feeling, and action systems" (Greenberg & Safron, 1984, p. 561).

The construct of *meaning system* is a three-dimensional schema for understanding the interaction among behavior, affect, and cognition. Meaning systems evolve from effective action (behavior) in the social environment and the individual's internal experience (cognitions, emotions) of that action. Meaning systems organize external with internal experience and continuously evolve via the interaction of the individual with the social domain.

The interdependence of the components of the meaning system enables the therapist to enter the client's meaning system through the component emphasized by the client. The altering of that one component through conversational exploration or the suggestion of a competing experience can shift the meaning system in its entirety, given the interaction among the components.

Recall Mark from Chapter 4, and the therapist's suggestion that Mark observe his concentration ability and how he was able at times to overcome his worry. The cognitive emphasis of the competing experience was based in Mark's description of the problem as primarily cognitive (i.e., concentration and worrying), rather than on an invariant focus on cognitions. Accepting Mark's emphasized component allowed the therapist entry into Mark's meaning system. Mark's cognitively altered experience of the problem permitted Mark to make new connections that ultimately led to not only an enhanced ability to concentrate, but also to an elimination of Mark's depression; the interaction among the components of the meaning system permitted not only cognitive changes, but also behavior and affective changes as well.

Common Theoretical Language

This theme points to the inherent problem that each orientation's jargon presents to eclectic endeavors (Goldfried & Newman, 1986). Gurman (1978) suggests that jargon impedes communication and calls for a common theoretical language to prevent the field from resembling a Tower of Babel.

While the need for a common unified theoretical language is a laudable goal, it is difficult to envision that any common language that arises from any particular orientation will be received with open arms. Translating one theory's constructs into the language of another theory or into a new meta-theory has not proven particularly fruitful. This is perhaps because there is so much historical and clinical richness embedded in each construct that such attempts lose something in the translation.

Rather than pursuing a common theoretical language through awkward translations or a new meta-theory that explains the diversity of all approaches, we propose a different perspective: A common theoretical language *can* be achieved if that language is the client's informal theory. The client's meaning system surrounding the presenting complaint is the common theoretical language and the framework from which therapy proceeds. We are suggesting that rather than attempting to develop a common theory, that instead the therapist accept the client's meaning system as the guiding theory from which to operate.

Each client presents the therapist with a new theory to learn and a different language to co-construct with the client. Emerging from the process of unfolding the client's meaning system, the therapist draws upon multiple models and adds to that process, leading to the cogeneration of a new theory or new meanings that permit the client to make the desired changes.

Rather than attempting awkward transformations that reduce the beauty and complexity of diverse approaches, we propose a process constructive theory that is nearly void of specific content so that the client's presented content can take precedence. The process nature of the theory permits the content to be co-constructed via the interaction between the therapist and the client. The process constructive theory is not a theory that attempts to translate all theories, or one that purports to explain or be meta to others, but rather it is an ever-changing chameleon that can reflect the elegant shade of insight perspectives as well as the pragmatic color of behaviorism. Although it contains its own jargon arising from the systems literature, the jargon of the theory recedes to the background once the client's content is introduced to the therapeutic process.

All the cases presented in this book illustrate the unique combination of ascending the client's language above the therapist's and the therapist and client constructing a common theoretical language. Recall Sandra from Chapter 4 and Hal from Chapter 7. Sandra's theoretical language was constructed as her depression's being related to her husband's impotency and the homeostatic function that both her depression and his impotence served in their marriage. Hal's theory emerged from the process to be that his depression was related to the dictatorship of his father and Hal's dissatisfaction with his job. Both cases exemplify taking the client's meaning system as the common theoretical language and through that process, constructing a theory that allows clients to meet their goals in therapy. The therapist contributes content from any of the rich sources of content made available through the ongoing acquisition of multiple ways of looking at client dilemmas.

Meta-Theoretical Principles of Change

This theme addresses the need to organize commonalities among successful therapists into a universal meta-theoretical set of principles of therapeutic change (Goldfried & Newman, 1986). The search for such a meta-theory of change arises from clinical and experimental evidence that the activities of experienced therapists are very similar, even though their conceptualizations are quite different (Sloane, Staples, Cristal, Yorkston, & Whipple, 1975).

The desire for meta-theoretical principles of change based upon successful therapies is congruent with Patterson's (1989) call for an eclectic approach based upon the common factors. The common factors, as will be discussed later, may already provide much of what is sought in such a meta theory. The same pitfalls, however, that befall a search for a common theoretical language can similarly obstruct the pursuit of universal principles of therapeutic change; that is, it is difficult, if not impossible, to incorporate the wide range of perspectives of how and why therapeutic change occurs in a unitary theory of change.

We proposed a multiple-level description of the change process. The multilevel description of change is not intended to account for or explain all views; it is not a unitary theory of change. Similar to the process constructive theory base, the multilevel description of change contains relatively little content so that it is but a skeleton or a general framework for understanding change. The therapist fills in the gaps with explanations of change from any theory he or she sees fit. The multilevel description is a pragmatic device to enable the therapist to pursue opportunities for change from a variety of perspectives.

Recall that the multilevel description presents change as a function of (1) interrupting the behavioral interaction that constitutes the problem cycle, (2) promoting meaning revision via the conversational recreation of the client's experience or the client's actual experience of the problem, and (3) the validation context provided by the therapist–client relationship. One may speculate that level one speaks to change from an action-oriented frame of reference (e.g., behavioral, structural, strategic), while level two addresses change from an internal processing level (e.g., cognitive, insight oriented), and level three from a humanistic perspective of the change process (e.g., client centered, Gestalt, existential). Such speculations, however valid on one level, are quite reductionistic on another level, and do not adequately reflect the complexity of the different approaches. We prefer to view the multilevel description as a pragmatic tool, rather than a universal model of change, leaving the therapist to select the explanation with which he or she is most comfortable. The multilevel view does not address change at a theoretical level, but rather at the clinical level of strategy.

Empirically Based Procedures

The final theme identified by Goldfried and Newman (1986) as important to eclecticism is an ideal long shared by researchers and clinicians across orientations: a theory of therapy and therapeutic procedures based on empirical foundations (Lazarus, 1971; Strupp, 1968).

This theme is readily apparent in the presented approach's emphasis on the psychotherapy outcome literature (Lambert et al., 1986). The outcome literature is extensive, covering decades, dealing with a wide range of clinical populations in diverse settings, and utilizing a variety of research designs (Lambert, 1986). Recall from Chapter 1 the percentages of outcome variance attributable to four therapeutic factors: Spontaneous remission accounts for 40% of outcome variance, common factors accounts for 30%, while placebo and specific technique each contribute to 15% of the variance.

The differential percentages of the four factors perfectly reflect their differential emphasis in the eclectic effort presented in this book. First and foremost, are those aspects of therapeutic improvement attributable to the client and the client's experience of out-of-therapy events (spontaneous remission). Simply put, the client is the most significant component of the change process.

Client specific variables that result in remission speak to clients' inherent resources and strengths, as well as their ability to utilize out-of-therapy events (e.g., social support, fortuitous events) as opportunities for change. Given that this factor is percentage-wise the most powerful, the therapeutic process may be viewed as an endeavor that creates a context that enables clients to access their own capacities for growth.

Accordingly, the presentation of the client and his or her meaning system regarding the presenting complaint, as well as the client's experience of between session events, always supersedes the therapist's agenda for any given session (our Pragmatic Assumption #2 speaks to spontaneous remission effects). The therapist should always be sensitive to spontaneous remission effects because, in our view, they are not really spontaneous, but rather a probable result of the inevitable responsiveness to variation provided by the psychotherapy context and the client's irrepressible tendencies toward health. All the interventions discussed in this book totally depend on the client's resources and ability to grow, as well as the ongoing nature of meaning revision outside of psychotherapy; competing experiences essentially attempt to empower spontaneous remission effects.

While spontaneous remission factors speak to the overwhelming significance of what the client brings to and experiences in therapy, common factors, the next most important variable with regard to outcome addresses what the therapist brings and the effects of the interpersonal system of the therapist–client relationship. Common factors (empathy, respect, genuineness), as perceived by the client, may account for most of the success gleaned from intervention (Lambert, 1986), and virtually all schools of therapy accept these relationship variables as significant to therapeutic progress (Patterson, 1989).

The common factors research, as well as the research specifically addressing the client's perception of the relationship (e.g., Bachelor, 1988; Gurman, 1977), encompasses the core element of the espoused approach. Pragmatic Assumption #1 speaks to common factors effects. The presented approach has attempted to maximize the effects of therapist-provided variables and empower relationship effects by expanding the definitions of empathy, respect, and genuineness while offering a method by which to extend the relationship context into the intervention process. The operationalization of common factors is discussed in detail later.

Last place in terms of significance to outcome is shared by placebo and specific technique factors. Placebo or expectancy effects include improvement that results from the client's knowledge of being in treatment, and consists of variables such as therapist credibility and the use of encouragement, persuasion, and reassurance (Lambert, 1986; Patterson, 1959). Lambert (1986) asserts that technical eclectic approaches that present a treatment with high credibility (e.g., relaxation) and a reasonable rationale (e.g., sympathetic overarousal) will be very powerful in mobilizing placebo effects. The selection of the content for conversation, as well as technique based upon the client's meaning system, explicitly addresses and, therefore, enhances client expectancies regarding therapy. Meeting the client's expectations regarding the goals and tasks of therapy would appear to enhance placebo effects by creating a cognitive set that expects change. Discussion of the applicability of a particular ascribed meaning or competing experience with a client may empower placebo by enhancing the intervention's credibility, as well as by conveying the therapist's encouragement and reassurance. Expectancy is also enhanced by the therapist's cognitive set, which conveys hope and expects change. If a client is perceived as difficult or unmotivated, the relationship may be adversely affected, and placebo will not be empowered. On the other hand, if the therapist perceives the client to be motivated and inherently capable of change, that attitude will be conveyed, and placebo will be enhanced.

Given the improvement in psychotherapy that results from client resources and strengths, fortuitous events, social support, common factors, and expectancy, there is consequently little room left for the clear demonstration of the research efficacy of specific techniques (Lambert, 1986). Nevertheless, there is some evidence of the usefulness of particular methods with particular problems, and it makes good clinical sense to consider the use of a demonstrated technique when confronted with a similar situation.

The eclectic approach presented in this book similarly recognizes the advantages of selecting research-tested techniques, but only if the techniques not only "match" the problem, but also are congruent with the client's meaning system regarding the problem. A selected technique must be seen as credible to the client and must fit the client's view of what is helpful.

Because technique only represents 15% of outcome variance, techniques are viewed only as formal content areas that may or may not prove useful in the unique circumstance of the client. For example, a couple may have erectile difficulties, and the therapist may select the intervention strategy of sensate focus (Masters & Johnson, 1970), based upon its demonstrated efficacy. However, if the clients do not see the applicability of the technique, or in their perception it seems similar to things they have tried before to no avail, then the demonstrated efficacy of sensate focus has little relevance, as well as little likelihood for success.

Eclecticism allows the therapist to survey the available literature and select interventions, as well as specific conceptualizations, to address clinical problems. Once selected, however, it seems that outcome depends far more on the client's resources and enactment of the technique, the therapist's style, attitude, and interpersonal relationship with the client, and the congruence of the technique with the client's meaning system.

By empowering spontaneous remission, operationalizing common factors, enhancing placebo, and discriminantly selecting technique, we have attempted to stack the cards of the outcome percentage game in favor of clients reaching their desired goals. Central to this attempt has been the interdependence of relationship and technique, and extending the common-factors context of the therapeutic relationship to the client's social environment by way of intervention strategies, that is, the operationalization of common factors.

OPERATIONALIZING COMMON FACTORS

Given the extensive literature supporting common factors, many have advocated their inclusion in all approaches, as well as their further study and operationalization. Two questions quickly come to mind: How can common factors be operationalized beyond therapist standby responses? How can the common-factors context of the therapist–client relationship become part of the intervention process itself?

This book has attempted to provide an answer to those questions and represents our proposal for operationalizing the common factors. The proposal began with the extension of the definitions of empathy, respect, and genuineness to include the client's perceptions and interpretations of the relationship and the values held by the therapist. An approach was advocated that viewed empathy as a function of the client's unique perceptions that required the therapist to respond flexibly to the client's empathic needs. Empathy was defined as therapists' attitudes and behaviors that place the client's perceptions and experiences above theoretical content and personal values; empathy is manifested by the therapist's attempts to not only accept and assume the internal frame of reference of the client (Rogers, 1951), but more important, also to *work within* the expressed meaning system of the client.

Respect was defined as attitudes and behaviors that place the value of the client as a person with worth and dignity above pejorative, pathological, or theoretical perspectives; respect is manifested by therapist sensitivity to the acceptability of any therapist behavior to the client's meaning system. Genuineness was defined as attitudes and behaviors that avoid phoniness and an overemphasis on authority (Cormier & Cormier, 1991) and embody an honest cautiousness regarding approaching the client, conceptualizing the client's concerns, and intervening to address those concerns. Genuineness is manifested by recognition of the client's expert status and an acceptance of the lack of definitive understanding provided by psychotherapy theory.

We proposed to operationalize common factors by first making the client's meaning system the theoretical orientation adopted by the therapist, thereby allowing the client's idiosyncratic experience of the world to become the guiding theory that dictates therapist behavior. The next step in operationalizing common factors was through what we called validation. Validation can be defined as a therapist-initiated process in which the client's thoughts, feelings, and behaviors are accepted, believed, and considered completely understandable given the client's subjective experience of the world. Validation reflects an individualized combination of the therapist variables of empathy, respect, and genuineness. The therapist genuinely accepts the client's presentation at face value, the therapist respects the client's experience of the problem by highlighting its importance, and the therapist empathically offers total justification of the client's experience. The therapist legitimizes the client's meaning system, and in the process may replace the invalidation that may be a part of it. Validation requires the therapist not only to accept the client's meaning system, but also to genuinely find a way to verbally convey the outright justification of the client's thoughts, feelings, and behaviors.

Common factors, as expressed through the acceptance of the client's meaning system as the guiding theory and the therapist's validation of that meaning system, provide the interpersonal context that creates meaning for any intervention. The common factors are further manifested by specific interventions that convey or implement the therapist's validation of the client's meaning system. Intervention may be effective to the extent that it validates the client's meaning system. Validation of the client's meaning system in the intervention process itself eliminates the artificial boundary between technique and relationship and extends the common factors context into the client's social environment.

Validation of the client's meaning system in the intervention process was discussed in Chapter 5 as occurring in two ways: (1) presenting the competing experience within a larger frame that validates the client's meaning system, and (2) designing the competing experience itself in such a way that it contains an inherent validation. Interventions are seen as explicit therapist behaviors that not only demonstrate empathy, respect, and genuineness, but also extend the relational context and its meaning of validation to the client's social environment. Such an extension is perhaps the most important aspect of encouraging clients to utilize their own strengths.

Our proposal devalues the significance of specific techniques and the standby therapist responses that usually come to mind when thinking of the common factors. Our proposal values how a specific technique emerges from the interpersonal system of the therapist–client relationship and how both technique and relationship interdependently provide a validation context, resting upon the meaning system of the client.

THE VALUES OF BRIEF THERAPY

Given that the presented approach purports to be committed to the values of efficiency and efficacy in clinical practice, Budman and Gurman's value ideals of a brief therapist may provide a useful method of evaluation. Rather than a point by point discussion of the eight ideals, we will summarize our own evaluation through the case examples presented in the book.

1. *"The brief therapist begins treatment by using the least radical procedure; that is, therapy begins with the least costly, least complicated, and least invasive treatment* (Budman & Gurman, 1988, p. 13). Recall Alice, David, and Jill, the 13-year-old who superficially cut her wrists and whom the parents described as overemotional. Rather than opting for intensive, weekly individual and family therapy or hospitalization to address this problem, the therapist only asked the parents to observe Jill and note the things they would like to see continue (de Shazer, 1985). Pursuing the least radical procedure led to termination in the second session. If no progress had been made or the situation had worsened, then another path could have been pursued.

2. *The brief therapist views cure as inconceivable* (Budman & Gurman, 1988, p. 17). Recall Lynn from Chapter 2 and her concern regarding her daughter's depression. The therapist addressed Lynn's concern about her daughter until Lynn no longer saw it as a problem. The therapist recognized that he could not (and didn't want to try to) change Lynn into a parent who would never be anxious or concerned again. Lynn reentered therapy 1 year later with concerns regarding her son's indecision about college.

3. *Brief therapists view people as malleable and as constantly changing and developing* (Budman & Gurman, 1988, p. 14). Recall Eric, Terry, and Michelle, who entered therapy because of Michelle's suicidal ideation. The therapist believed that although the family was temporarily stuck and at a low creative ebb, that ultimately all the individuals were in the process of moving beyond the current crisis. The family's presentation was only a snapshot of an ongoing developmental and transitional sequence.

Minimal therapeutic intervention enabled an opportunity for the family to move beyond the presenting snapshot of restricted options and a suicidal adolescent.

4. *The brief therapist, while maintaining an appreciation for the role of psychiatric diagnosis, has a health, rather than illness, orientation* (Budman & Gurman, 1988). Recall Richard, who appeared as very hostile and guarded, and who suspected his wife of having an affair. While consideration of the diagnostic category of paranoia and the information that it yields was ever present in the therapist's mind, the diagnostic information gave way as the therapeutic conversation unfolded enough to present another avenue of intervention to pursue. The more the dialogue progressed, the more Richard's resources became apparent. If Richard had remained hostile and held rigidly to all his behaviors and beliefs regarding his wife's affair, then the role of psychiatric diagnosis may have proven helpful.

5. *The brief therapist takes the patient's presenting problem seriously and hopes to help make changes in some areas that the patient specifies or comes to clarify as important* (Budman & Gurman, 1988, p. 14). Recall Joe, who presented as a messenger from God. The therapist accepted at face value Joe's problem in spreading God's Word and intervened to help Joe make changes in his methods, because it was an area that Joe specified as important. Respecting what the client clarifies as important enables a process that encourages further client change and growth. Joe eventually returned to college and pursued a major in religion.

6. *The brief therapist realizes that he or she may not be thanked for changes that have occurred after therapy, and may not, after relatively few visits, ever see the patient again* (Budman & Gurman, 1988, p. 14). Recall Monte from Chapter 6, whose greatest fear was that he would end up hopelessly mentally ill and institutionalized like his father. Monte suffered from panic attacks nearly every day for the previous 2 years before entering therapy. The therapist, after following a variety of avenues, suggested a symptom prescription. Monte returned having had no panic attacks *and* reporting that he had quit smoking. Monte took full responsibility for the change (rightfully so) and did not acknowledge the therapist or psychotherapy as being helpful. The therapist has had no further contact.

7. *The brief therapist assumes that psychotherapy may be "for better or for worse" and that not everyone who requests treatment needs or can benefit from it* (Budman & Gurman, 1988, p. 15). This ideal represents our only point of contention with Budman and Gurman's (1988) value ideals. While we wholeheartedly agree that psychotherapy can be for better or worse, we also believe that those *requesting* treatment have every right to have a therapist attempt to address their needs. This is not to say that some clients will not benefit from therapy or will not present special challenges to the therapist. Rather, we prefer to err on the side of attempting to allow

things to unfold and see what happens, as opposed to categorically dismissing certain clients or determining a client to be addicted to therapy on an a priori basis.

8. *Being in the world is seen as far more important than being in therapy* (Budman & Gurman, 1988, p. 15). Recall Hal, whose self-ascribed loser self-image, job dissatisfaction, and dependence on his father resulted in an understandable depression. Although Hal's past was discussed, validated, and connected to his current depressed state, the focus of therapy was Hal's present problems and ongoing relationships, and how he was going to address them. Such a focus reflects a perspective that attempts to create opportunities for meaningful change to enable clients to get on with their lives and get out of therapy. In the termination session, Hal expressed a similar view when he jokingly commented on his guilt about being in therapy instead of studying; being in the world became primary over being in therapy.

CONCLUSIONS

It has not been our intent to propose the definitive model of eclectic individual and family therapy; neither has our interest been to present a model at all. Rather, we have attempted to share some of the evolving meanings that we have ascribed to the psychotherapeutic process that are currently organizing our perceptions and experiences regarding the practice of therapy. We do not want to add to the 250-plus available models, but rather seek to provide input to therapists who are thinking about their work as therapists and struggling to revise their clinical work toward more flexibility.

Although the presented approach cannot be afforded the status of a model, we believe that it does offer a step in the right direction on three different paths. The first path leads to a wellness point of view, as opposed to just another repair strategy based in deficit and dysfunction. It is likely obvious to the reader where we stand regarding models of psychopathology and the diagnosis of mental disorders. Our stance is not original, nor is our emphasis on idiographic views versus nomethetic views of human functioning (e.g., Allport, 1937; Garfield, 1957, 1983). The major problem we have with diagnosis and pathology is a pragmatic one. We simply fail to see its relevance *most* of the time in terms of addressing people in distress or empowering a context that allows people to change.

The second path is one that leads to a "pure" process description of psychotherapy that permits the various theoretical descriptions of etiology and treatment to remain rich and separate. Rather than a definitive, all-encompassing description of psychotherapy that provides an inherently right way to practice, such a process view would provide just enough structure and guidance to help clinicians tolerate the uncertainty of face-to-face meetings with people in pain. We believe that while there is a long way to go on this path, a process constructive therapy base is one step in the right direction, and we look for other process-oriented views to continue to emerge.

The final path is one that leads to the operationalization of common factors beyond global generalities about empathic relationships to specific ways of making relationship effects become manifest. This includes removing the arbitrary distinction between relationship and technique (Butler & Strupp, 1986) and emphasizing more the client's interpretation about the relationship. Common factors may not be understood apart from the therapeutic context; it is the interface of human interaction that provides them with definition. Consequently, definitions will vary from individual to individual and interaction to interaction.

It has long been debated whether or not the therapist provided variables are necessary *and* sufficient to promote therapeutic change. While all advocate their necessity, many question the degree to which the variables are sufficient. In many ways, we believe that the common factors *are* sufficient and that it is perhaps their definition and operationalization that has been insufficient to account for the diversity of client interpersonal styles in therapy.

References

Alexander, L. B., & Luborsky, L. (1986). The Penn helping alliance scales. In L. S. Greenberg & W. M. Pinsof (Eds.), *The psychotherapeutic process: A research handbook* (pp. 325–366). New York: Guilford Press.

Allport, G. W. (1937). *Personality: A psychological interpretation.* New York: Henry Holt.

Anderson, H., & Goolishian, H. (1988). Human systems as linguistic systems: Preliminary and evolving ideas about the implications for clinical theory. *Family Process, 27,* 371–393.

Asch, Solomon E. (1946). Forming impressions of personality. *Journal of Abnormal and Social Psychology, 41,* 258.

Bachelor, A. (1988). How clients perceive therapist empathy. *Psychotherapy, 25,* 227–240.

Bachelor, A. (1991). Comparison and relationship to outcome of diverse dimensions of the helping alliance as seen by client and therapist. *Psychotherapy, 28,* 534–549.

Bandura, A., Blanchard, E. B., & Ritter, B. (1969). The relative efficacy of desensitization and modeling approaches for inducing behavioral, affective, and cognitive changes. *Journal of Personality and Social Psychology, 13,* 173–199.

Barlow, D. H. (1988). *Anxiety and its disorders.* New York: Guilford.

Barlow, D. H., & Wolfe, B. (1981). Behavioral approaches to anxiety disorders. *Journal of Consulting and Clinical Psychology, 49,* 448–454.

Barrett-Lennard, G. T. (1981). The empathy cycle: Refinement of a nuclear concept. *Journal of Counseling Psychology, 28,* 91–100.

Bateson, G. (1955). A theory of play and fantasy. *APA Psychiatric Research Reports, 2,* 177–193.

Bateson, G., Jackson, D. D., Haley, J., & Weakland, J. (1956). Toward a theory of schizophrenia. *Behavioral Science, 1,* 251–264.

Beauchamp, J. F., & Childress, R. F. (1983). *Principles of biomedical ethics* (2nd ed.). New York: Oxford University Press.

Beauvoir, S. de (1953). *The second sex* (H. M. Parshley, Trans., & Ed.). New York: Knopf.

Bergin, A. E. (1971). The evaluation of therapeutic outcome. In A. E. Bergin & S. L. Garfield (Eds.), *Handbook of psychotherapy and behavior change* (pp. 217–270). New York: Wiley.

Bergin, A. E. & Lambert, M. J. (1978). The evaluation of therapeutic outcomes. In S. L. Garfield & A. E. Bergin (Eds.), *Handbook of psychotherapy and behavior change* (2nd ed., pp. 139–190). New York: Wiley.

Beutler, L. E. (1983). *Eclectic psychotherapy: A systematic approach.* New York: Pergamon Press.

Beutler, L. E. (1986). Systematic eclectic psychotherapy. In J. C. Norcross (Ed.), *Handbook of eclectic psychotherapy* (pp. 94–131). New York: Brunner/Mazel.

Bodin, A. M. (1981). The interactional view: Family therapy approaches of the Mental Research Institute. In A. S. Gurman & D. P. Kniskern (Eds.), *Handbook of family therapy* (pp. 267–311). New York: Brunner/Mazel.

Bok, S. (1978). *Lying: A moral choice in public and private life* (1st ed.). New York: Pantheon Books.

Bordin, E. S. (1979). The generalizability of the psychoanalytic concept of the working alliance. *Psychotherapy, 16,* 252–260.

Buckley, W. (1967). *Sociology and modern systems theory.* Englewood Cliffs, NJ: Prentice-Hall.

Budman, S. H., & Gurman, A. S. (1988). *Theory and practice of brief therapy.* New York: Guilford Press.

Burgess, A. W., & Holmstrom, L. L. (1979). *Rape: Crisis and recovery.* Bowie, MD: Robert J. Brady.

Butcher, J. N., & Koss, M. P. (1978). Research on brief and crisis-oriented therapies. In S. Garfield & A. E. Bergin (Eds.), *Handbook of psychotherapy and behavior change* (2nd ed., pp. 725–768). New York: Wiley.

Butler, S. F., & Strupp, H. H. (1986). Specific and nonspecific factors in psychotherapy: A problematic paradigm for psychotherapy research. *Psychotherapy, 23,* 30–40.

Carkhuff, R. R. (1971). *The development of human resources.* New York: Holt, Rinehart & Winston.

Cormier, W. H., & Cormier, L. S. (1991). *Interviewing strategies for helpers* (3rd ed.). Pacific Grove, CA: Brooks/Cole.

Corsini, R. J. (1981). *Handbook of innovative psychotherapies* New York: Wiley.

Coyne, J. C. (1986). The significance of the interview in strategic marital therapy. *Journal of Strategic and Systemic Therapies, 5,* 63–70.

Cronen, V. E., Johnson, K. M., & Lannamann, J. W. (1982). Paradoxes, double binds, and reflexive loops. *Family Process, 21,* 91–112.

Davison, G. C., & Neale, J. M. (1986). *Abnormal psychology.* New York: Wiley.

Dell, P. (1981). Paradox redux. *Journal of Marital and Family Therapy, 7,* 127–134.

de Shazer, S. (1985). *Keys to solutions in brief therapy.* New York: W. W. Norton.

de Shazer, S., Berg, I., Lipchik, E., Nunnolly, E., Molnar, A., Gingerich, W., & Weiner-Davis, M. (1986). Brief therapy: Focused solution development. *Family Process, 25,* 207–222.

Driscoll, R. (1984). *Pragmatic psychotherapy.* New York: Van Nostrand Reinhold.

Duncan, B. L. (1984). Adopting the construct of functionality when it facilitates system change: A method of selective integration. *Journal of Strategic and Systemic Therapies, 4,* 58–63.

Duncan, B. L. (1989). Paradoxical procedures in family therapy. In M. Ascher (Ed.), *Therapeutic paradox* (pp. 310–348). New York: Guilford.

Duncan, B. L. (1992a). Strategic therapy, eclecticism, and the therapeutic relationship. *Journal of Marital and Family Therapy, 18,* 17–23.

Duncan, B. L. (1992b). Strategy and reality: A reply to Held, Goolishian, and Anderson. *Journal of Marital and Family Therapy, 18,* 39–40.

Duncan, B. L. (in press). Creating opportunities for rapid change in marital therapy. In R. A. Wells & V. J. Gianetti (Eds.), *Casebook of the brief psychotherapies.* New York: Plenum.

Duncan, B. L., & Fraser, J. S. (1987). Buckley's scheme of schemes as a foundation for teaching family systems theory. *Journal of Marital and Family Therapy, 13,* 299–305.

Duncan, B. L., & Parks, M. B. (1988). Integrating individual and systems approaches: Strategic-behavioral therapy. *Journal of Marital and Family Therapy, 14,* 151–161.

Duncan, B. L., Parks, M. B., & Rusk, G. S. (1990). Eclectic strategic practice: A process constructive perspective. *Journal of Marital and Family Therapy, 16,* 165–178.

Duncan, B. L., & Rock, J. W. (1991). *Overcoming relationship impasses: Ways to initiate change when your partner won't help.* New York: Insight Books.

Duncan, B. L., Rock, J. W., & Parks, M. B. (1987). Strategic-behavioral therapy: A practical alternative. *Psychotherapy, 24,* 192–202.

Duncan, B. L., & Solovey, A. (1989). Strategic brief therapy: An insight-oriented approach? *Journal of Marital and Family Therapy, 15,* 1–9.

Emery, G., & Campbell, J. (1986). *Rapid relief from emotional distress.* New York: Rawson Associates.

Erickson, M. H. (1980). Collected papers. In E. L. Rossi (Ed.), *Collected papers of Milton Erickson.* New York: Irvington.

Fisch, R., Weakland, J., & Segal, L. (1982). *The tactics of change: Doing therapy briefly.* San Francisco: Jossey-Bass.

Frank, J. D. (1973). *Persuasion and healing* (2nd ed.), Baltimore: The Johns Hopkins University Press.

Frank, J. D. (1982). Therapeutic components shared by all psychotherapies. In J. H. Harvey & M. M. Peeks (Eds.), *Psychotherapy research and behavior change* (pp. 9–37). Washington, DC: American Psychological Association.

Fraser, J. S. (1984a). Process level integration: Corrective vision for a binocular view. *Journal of Strategic and Systemic Therapies, 4,* 43–57.

Fraser, J. S. (1984b). Paradox or orthodox: Folie a deux? *Journal of Marital and Family Therapy, 10,* 361–372.

Fraser, J. S. (1986). Integrating system-based therapies: Similarities, differences, and some critical questions. In D. E. Efron (Ed.), *Journeys: Expansion of the strategic-systemic therapies* (pp. 125–149). New York: Brunner/Mazel.

Garfield, S. L. (1957). *Introductory clinical psychology.* New York: Macmillan.

Garfield, S. L. (1971). Research on client variables in psychotherapy. In A. E. Bergin & S. Garfield (Eds.), *Handbook of psychotherapy and behavior change* (pp. 271–298). New York: Wiley.

Garfield, S. L. (1978). Research on client variables in psychotherapy. In S. L. Garfield & A. E. Bergin (Eds.), *Handbook of psychotherapy and behavior change* (2nd ed., pp. 191–232). New York: Wiley.

Garfield, S. L. (1983). *Clinical psychology. The study of personality and behavior.* (Revised ed). Hawthorne, NY: Aldine.

Garfield, S. L. (1986). An eclectic psychotherapy. In J. C. Norcross (Ed.), *Handbook of eclectic psychotherapy* (pp. 132–162). New York: Brunner/Mazel.

Garfield, S. L., & Kurtz, R. (1977). A study of eclectic views. *Journal of Consulting and Clinical Psychology, 45,* 78–83.

Gergen, K. J. (1985). The social constructionist movement in modern psychology. *American Psychologist, 40,* 266–275.

Gilder, G. (1987). *Men and marriage.* Los Angeles: Pelican.

Goldfried, M. R., & Newman, C. (1986). Psychotherapy integration: An historical perspective. In J. C. Norcross (Ed.), *Handbook of eclectic psychotherapy* (pp. 25–64). New York: Brunner/Mazel.

Goldfried, M. R., & Safran, J. D. (1986). Future directions in psychotherapy integration. In J. B. Norcross (Ed.), *Handbook of eclectic psychotherapy* (pp. 463–484). New York: Brunner/Mazel.

Goolishian, H., & Anderson, H. (1987). Language systems and therapy: An evolving idea. *Psychotherapy, 24,* 529–538.

Goolishian, H., & Anderson, H. (1992). Strategy and intervention versus non-intervention: A matter of theory. *Journal of Marital and Family Therapy, 18,* 5–15.

Green, S. L., & Hansen, J. C. (1989). Ethical dilemmas faced by family therapists. *Journal of Marital and Family Therapy, 15,* 149–158.

Greenberg, L. S., & Safran, J. D. (1984). Integrating affect and cognitions: A perspective on the process of therapeutic change. *Cognitive Therapy and Research, 8,* 559–578.

Gurman, A. S. (1977). Therapist and patient factors influencing the patient's perception of facilitative therapeutic conditions. *Psychiatry, 40,* 16–24.

Gurman, A. S. (1978). Contemporary marital therapies: A critique and comparative analysis of psychodynamic, behavioral and systems theory approaches. In T. Paolino & B. McCrady (Eds.), *Marriage and marital therapy* (pp. 445–566). New York: Brunner/Mazel.

Gurman, A. S., & Kniskern, D. P. (1978). Research on marital and family therapy: Progress, perspective, and prospect. In S. L. Garfield & A. E. Bergin (Eds.), *Handbook of psychotherapy and behavior change* (2nd ed., pp. 817–902). New York: Wiley.

Gurman, A. S., Kniskern, D. P., & Pinsof, W. M. (1986). Research on the process and outcome of marital and family therapy. In S. L. Garfield & A. E. Bergin (Eds.), *Handbook of psychotherapy and behavior change* (3rd ed., pp. 565–626). New York: Wiley.

Haley, J. (1984). *Ordeal therapy.* San Francisco: Jossey-Bass.

Haley, J. (1987). *Problem solving therapy* (2nd ed.). San Francisco: Jossey-Bass.

Hare-Mustin, R. T. (1987). The problem of gender in family therapy theory. *Family Process, 26,* 15–27.

Hare-Mustin, R. T., & Maracek, J. (Eds.). (1990). *Making a difference: Psychology and the construction of gender.* New Haven: Yale University Press.

Hartley, D., & Strupp, H. (1983). The therapeutic alliance: Its relationship to outcome in brief psychotherapy. In J. Masling (Ed.), *Empirical studies of psychoanalytic theories* (Vol. 1, pp. 1–27). Hillsdale, NJ: Erlbaum.

Heath, A. W., & Atkinson, B. J. (1989). Solutions attempted and considered: Broadening assessment in brief therapy. *Journal of Strategic and Systemic Therapies, 8,* 56–57.

Held, B. S. (1984). Toward a strategic eclecticism: A proposal. *Psychotherapy, 21,* 232–241.

Held, B. S. (1986). The relationship between individual psychologies and strategic/systemic therapies reconsidered. In D. E. Efron (Ed.), *Journeys: Expansion of the strategic systemic therapies* (pp. 222–260). New York: Brunner/Mazel.

Held, B. S. (1991). The process/content distinction in psychotherapy revisited. *Psychotherapy, 28,* 207–217.

Hoffman, L. (1985). Beyond power and control: Toward a second-order family systems therapy. *Family Systems Medicine, 3,* 381–396.

Horvath, A. O., & Greenberg, L. (1986). Development and validation of the Working Alliance Inventory. *Journal of Counseling Psychology, 36,* 223–233.

Jackson, D., & Lederer, W. (1968). *The mirages of marriage.* New York: W. W. Norton.

Johnson, D. W. (1981). *Reaching out: Interpersonal effectiveness and self-actualization.* Englewood Cliffs, NJ: Prentice-Hall.

Koss, M. P. (1979). Length of psychotherapy for clients seen in private practice. *Journal of Consulting and Clinical Psychology, 47,* 210–212.

Koss, M. P., & Butcher, J. N. (1986). Research on brief psychotherapy. In S. L. Garfield & A. E. Bergin (Eds.), *Handbook of psychotherapy and behavior change* (3rd ed., pp. 627–670). New York: Wiley.

Kubler-Ross, E. (1969). *On death and dying.* New York: Macmillan.

Kuehl, B. P., Newfield, N. A., & Joanning, H. (1990). A client-based description of family therapy. *Journal of Family Psychology, 3,* 310–321.

LaCrosse, M. B. (1980). Perceived counselor social influence and counseling outcomes: Validity of the Counselor Rating Form. *Journal of Counseling Psychology, 27,* 320–327.

Lambert, M. (1986). Implications of psychotherapy outcome research for eclectic psychotherapy. In J. C. Norcross (Ed.), *Handbook of eclectic psychotherapy* (pp. 436–462). New York: Brunner/Mazel.

Lambert, M. J., Shapiro, D. A., & Bergin, A. E. (1986). The effectiveness of psychotherapy. In S. L. Garfield & A. E. Bergin (Eds.), *Handbook of psychotherapy and behavior change* (3rd ed., pp. 157–212). New York: Wiley.

Langsley, D. G. (1978). Comparing clinic and private practice of psychiatry. *American Journal of Psychiatry, 135,* 702–706.

Lazarus, A. A. (1967). In support of technical eclecticism. *Psychological Reports, 21,* 415–416.

Lazarus, A. A. (1971). *Behavior therapy and beyond.* New York: McGraw-Hill.

Lazarus, A. A. (1981). *The practice of multimodal therapy.* New York: McGraw-Hill.

Luborsky, L., Chandler, M., Auerbach, A. H., Cohen, J., & Bachrach, H. A. (1971). Factors influencing the outcome of psychotherapy: A review of quantitative research. *Psychological Bulletin, 75,* 145–185.

Luborsky, L., Crits-Christoph, P., Alexander, L., Margolis, M., & Cohen, M. (1983). Two helping alliance methods of predicting outcomes of psychotherapy. *Journal of Nervous and Mental Disease, 171,* 480–491.

Luborsky, L., Singer, B., & Luborsky, L. (1975). Comparative studies of psychotherapies. *Archives of General Psychiatry, 32,* 995–1008.

MacKinnon, L. K., & Miller, D. (1987). The new epistemology and the Milan approach: Feminism and sociopolitical considerations. *Journal of Marital and Family Therapy. 13*, 139–155.

Madanes, C. (1981). *Strategic family therapy*. San Francisco: Jossey-Bass.

Madanes, C. (1990). *Sex, love, and violence*. New York: W. W. Norton.

Marziali, E. (1984). Three viewpoints on the therapeutic alliance: Similarities, differences, and associations with psychotherapy outcome. *Journal of Nervous and Mental Diseases, 172*, 417–423.

Masters, W. H., & Johnson, V. E. (1970). *Human sexual inadequacy*. Boston: Little Brown.

Matarazzo, J. (1965). Psychotherapeutic processes. *Annual Review of Psychology, 16*, 181–224.

Norcross, J. C. (1986). Eclectic psychotherapy. In J.C. Norcross (Ed.), *Handbook of eclectic psychotherapy* (pp. 3–24). New York: Brunner/Mazel.

Norcross, J. C. (1991). Prescriptive matching in psychotherapy: An introduction. *Psychotherapy, 28*, 439–483.

O'Hanlon, W. H., & Weiner-Davis, M. (1989). *In search of solutions*. New York: W. W. Norton.

O'Hanlon, W. H., & Wilk, J. (1987). *Shifting contexts*. New York: Guilford Press.

Orlinsky, D. E., & Howard, K. I. (1986). Process and outcome in psychotherapy. In S. L. Garfield & A. E. Bergin (Eds.), *Handbook of psychotherapy and behavior change* (3rd ed., pp. 311–381). New York: Wiley.

Park, B., & Rothbart, M. (1982). Perception of out-group homogeneity and levels of social categorization: Memory for the subordinate attributes of in-group and out-group members. *Journal of Personality and Social Psychology, 42*, 1051–1068.

Parry, A. (1991). A universe of stories. *Family Process, 30*, 37–54.

Patterson, C. H. (1959). *Counseling and psychotherapy: Theory and Practice*. New York: Harper & Row.

Patterson, C. H. (1984). Empathy, warmth, and genuineness in psychotherapy: A review of reviews. *Psychotherapy, 21*, 431–438.

Patterson, C. H. (1989). Foundations for a systematic eclectic psychotherapy. *Psychotherapy, 26*, 427–435.

Pinsof, W. M. (1983). Integrative problem-centered therapy: Toward the synthesis of family and individual psychotherapies. *Journal of Marital and Family Therapy, 9*, 19–35.

Pinsof, W. M., & Catherall, D. R. (1986). The integrative psychotherapy alliance: Family, couple, and individual scale. *Journal of Marital and Family Therapy, 12*, 137–151.

Prochaska, J. O. (1991). Prescribing to the stage and level of phobia patients. *Psychotherapy, 28*, 463–468.

Prochaska, J. O., & DiClemente, C. C. (1982). Transtheoretical therapy: Toward a more integrative model of change. *Psychotherapy, 19*, 276–288.

Prochaska, J. O., & DiClemente, C. C. (1984). *The transtheoretical approach*. Homewood, IL: Dow Jones/Irwin.

Redd, W. H., Porterfield, A. L., & Anderson, B. L. (1979). *Behavior modification: Behavioral approaches to human problems*. New York: Random House.

Rogers, C. R. (1951). *Client-centered therapy*. Boston: Houghton Mifflin.

Rogers, C. R. (1957). The necessary and sufficient conditions of therapeutic personality change. *Journal of Consulting Psychology, 21*, 95–103.

Rohrbaugh, M., & Eron, J. B. (1982). The strategic systems therapies. In L. E. Abt & I. R. Stuart (Eds.), *The newer therapies: A workbook* (pp. 152–194). New York: Van Nostrand Reinhold.

Rosenbaum, R. (1990). Strategic psychotherapy. In R. A. Wells & V. J. Grannetti (Eds.), *Handbook of the brief psychotherapies* (pp. 351–404). New York: Plenum Press.

Rosenfield, I. (1988). *The invention of memory.* New York: Basic.

Rosenhan, D. L. (1984). On being sane in insane places. In P. Watzlawick (Ed.), *The invented reality* (pp. 117–144). New York: W. W. Norton.

Rubinstein, E. A., & Lorr, M. (1956). A comparison of terminators and remainers in out-patient psychotherapy. *Journal of Clinical Psychology, 12,* 345–349.

Saltzman, N., & Norcross, J. C. (Eds.). (1990). *Therapy wars.* San Francisco: Jossey-Bass.

Schwartz, R. (1989). Maybe there is a better way: Response to Duncan and Solovey. *Journal of Marital and Family Therapy, 11–12,* 13–16.

Schwartz, R. M. (1982). Cognitive–behavior modification: A conceptual review. *Clinical Psychology Review, 2,* 267–293.

Selvini, M. (Ed.) (1988). *The work of Mara Selvini-Palazzoli.* Northvale, NJ: Jason Aronson.

Selvini-Palazzoli, M., Boscolo, L., Cecchin, G., & Prata, G. (1978). *Paradox and counterparadox.* New York: Jason Aronson.

Selvini-Palazzoli, M. (1986). Toward a general model of psychotic family games. *Journal of Marital and Family Therapy, 12,* 339–349.

Shafer, R. (1983). *The analytic attitude.* New York: Basic.

Slipp, S. (1989). A different viewpoint for integrating psychodynamic and systems approaches. *Journal of Marital and Family Therapy, 15,* 13–16.

Sloane, R. B., Staples, F. R., Cristol, A. H., Yorkston, N. J., & Whipple, K. (1975). *Psychotherapy versus behavior therapy.* Cambridge, MA: Harvard University Press.

Smith, M. L., Glass, G. V., & Miller, T. I. (1980). *The benefits of psychotherapy.* Baltimore: Johns Hopkins University Press.

Solovey, A. D., & Duncan, B. L. (1992). Ethics and strategic therapy: A proposed ethical direction. *Journal of Marital and Family Therapy, 18,* 53–61.

Spence, D. P. (1984). *Narrative truth and historical truth.* New York: W. W. Norton.

Stanton, M. D. (1981). Strategic approaches to family therapy. In A. S. Gurman & D. P. Kniskern (Eds.), *Handbook of family therapy* (pp. 361–402). New York: Brunner/Mazel.

Strupp, H. H. (1968). Psychotherapists and (or versus?) researchers. *Voices: The art and science of psychotherapy, 4,* 28–37.

Truax, C. B., & Carkhuff, R. R. (1967). *Toward effective counseling and psychotherapy.* Chicago: Aldine.

Ullman, L. P., & Krasner, L. (1975). *A psychological approach to abnormal behavior* (2nd ed.). Englewood Cliffs, NJ: Prentice-Hall.

Varela, F. J. (1989). Reflections on the circulation of concepts between a biology of cognition and systemic family therapy. *Family Process, 28,* 15–24.

Wachtel, P. L. (1977). *Psychoanalysis and behavior therapy: Toward an integration.* New York: Basic Books.

Walsh, F., & Scheinkman, M. (1989). (Fe)male: The hidden gender dimension in models of family therapy. In M. McGoldrick, C. Anderson, & F. Walsh (Eds.),

Women in families: A framework for family therapy (pp. 16–41). New York: W. W. Norton.

Waterson, J. A., Gallessich, J. M., & Hanson, G. R. (1987). *Family therapists' ethical concerns regarding the use of paradoxical techniques.* Unpublished manuscript.

Watzlawick, P. (1984). *The invented reality.* New York: W. W. Norton.

Watzlawick, P., Beavin, J., & Jackson, D. D. (1967). *The pragmatics of human communication.* New York: W. W. Norton.

Watzlawick, P., Weakland, J., & Fisch, R. (1974). *Change: Principles of problem formation and problem resolution.* New York: W. W. Norton.

Weakland, J. H., Fisch, R., Watzlawick, P., & Bodin, A. (1974). Brief therapy: Focused problem resolution. *Family Process, 13,* 141–168.

Wegner, D. M., Vallacher, R. R., Macomber, G., Wood, R., & Arps, K. (1984). The emergence of action. *Journal of Personality and Social Psychology, 46,* 269–279.

Weiner, I. B. (1975). *Principles of psychotherapy.* New York: Wiley.

Weitzman, L. J. (1985). *The divorce revolution: The unexpected social and economic consequences for women and children in America.* New York: Free Press.

Wendorf, D. J., & Wendorf, R. J. (1985). A systemic view of family therapy ethics. *Family Process, 4,* 443–453.

Wiesel, E. (1966). *The gates of the forest.* New York: Schocken Books.

Wilden, A. (1972). *System and structure: Essays in communication and exchange.* London: Tavistock.

Wilson, R. (1986). *Don't panic. Taking control of anxiety attacks.* New York: Harper & Row.

Appendix A

Interventions

T HE following interventions are a compilation of strategies (competing experiences) from a variety of sources that may be utilized to promote revision experiences. They were chosen because of their exceptional utility and because they come from a literature base to which many therapists have not been exposed. The source title, author, and page number are listed for convenient reference. The interventions are briefly described to enable the reader to determine the general client descriptions in which they may be considered. Many of these interventions were exemplified in this volume and are indicated by an asterisk.

Source	Intervention	Description/ appropriate situation
Keys to Solutions in Brief Therapy (de Shazer, 1985) p. 122	"Do Something Different": Between now and the next time we meet, I would like each of you once, to do something different when (the problem occurs)."	Formula task for any situation in which client(s) seem stuck in rut. Acesses clients' creative capacities.
p. 81	"Crystal Ball Technique"* (miracle question): If a miracle occurred overnight and the problem disappeared, what will things be like for you and others?	Formula task for any situation. Contructs expectations for the future without the problem. A vision of the future can become a reality.
p. 132	"Overcoming"*: "Pay attention to what you do when you overcome the urge (temptation) to (eat, drink, feel depressed, yell at spouse, etc.)."	Formula task for any situation in which clients present a problem about themselves. Enables the experience of exceptions

		to the problem that may be amplified.
p. 137	"First Session Formula Task"*: "Between now and next time we meet, observe so that you can describe what happens in your (life, relationship, child) that you would like to continue to have happen.	Formula task for any situation. Shifts focus from past to present and future and promotes expectations of change. Encourages the notation of exceptions that may be amplified.
Family Process (de Shazer et al., 1986) p. 213	"Rate and Predict"*: "Before going to bed, predict your rate of (depression, anxiety, etc.) on a scale of 1–10, for the following day. The next night, and thereafter, record your actual rate for the day and then compare your actual versus predicted rate. Note any differences and consider what the differences are about.	Formula task for any situation in which clients present a problem about themselves. Encourage clients to note exceptions as well as the connection between what they do and how they experience the problem.
Tactics of Change (Fisch, Weakland, & Segal, 1982) p. 129	"Attempting to Force Something That Can Only Occur Spontaneously": The therapist designs a task that implicitly asks clients to alter their problem by performing another behavior that is mutually exclusive. (Client with erectile difficulty asked to intentionally lose erection and explore thoughts and feelings during actual experience.)	Useful in addressing human performance problems (erectile difficulties, sleep problems, orgasmic difficulties). Helps client give up self-coercive attempts to correct problem by giving instructions to fail in the performance.
p. 136	"Attempting to Master a Feared Event by Postponing It"*: The therapist designs a task that exposes the client to the feared task, while restraining the client from success-	

	fully completing it. (Client with driving phobia asked to start car and drive no more than to the end of the driveway.)	Useful for clients attempting to solve a problem by avoiding the situation (phobias, writing blocks, shyness, etc.). The client is exposed to the feared event in a way that requires nonmastery.
p. 159	"Go Slow" The client is instructed to do little or nothing about the problem; therapist provides valid rationales for going slowly in terms of resolving the problem.	Useful for clients trying too hard to resolve a problem or are pressing the therapist for immediate answers. Go slow removes sense of urgency and enables clients to relax problem-maintaining solutions. Often a welcomed relief accompanies the therapist's suggestion to "go slowly."
p. 162	"Dangers of Improvement"*: Clients are asked to recognize the dangers inherent in resolving the problem.	Useful for clients who are ambivalent about change or who have struggled with making a change for a long time. Validates difficulties inherent to change, allowing client to move beyond being stuck by them.

Tactics of Change also presents several other interventions, including: "Attempting to Reach Accord Through Opposition," "Confirming the Accuser's Suspicions by Defending Oneself," and "Demanding Compliance Through Voluntarism." The intervention names are descriptive of client solutions to the problem.

Ordeal Therapy (Haley, 1984)	"The Ordeal Technique"*: The therapist designs an ordeal that essentially attaches a negative, but productive consequence to a client's symptom. (Client asked to clean house for minimum of

	30 minutes when symptom occurs.)	Useful for interrupting solution attempts and to motivate clients to act, rather than think about problem.
Sex, Love, and Violence (Madanes, 1990) p. 26	"Prescribing the Symptom"": Clients are asked to engage in or encourage the problem. Parents may be encouraged to prescribe a symptom to a child.	Useful as a way of allowing clients to take control of behavior that seems out of control. Creates opportunities for control or spaces in which symptom is not occurring.
p. 29	"Prescribing a Symbolic Act" Clients are asked to perform repetitively an act that is symbolic of a self-destructive act, but that lacks the self-destructive consequences. (Bulimic client asked to buy favorite foods, mush it up, and throw down the toilet.)	Useful for self- destructive behaviors. Madanes believes self-destructive acts are attempts to punish those who are perceived as not providing enough love.
p. 31	"Prescribing the Pretending of the Symptom" Clients (adults and children) are asked to pretend to have the symptom and significant others are asked to comfort as per usual.	Useful for a variety of situations, but especially with child symptoms. Madanes believes that a child's problems express a problem of the parents. Introduces play into problem pattern. Can be combined with observe task: Client asked to periodically pretend to have problem, and significant others to observe and figure out when it's real or pretend.

Sex, Love, and Violence also presents several other interventions, including "Sixteen Steps to Reparation in Cases of Sexual Abuse," a very useful framework for family recovery from sexual abuse.

The Work of Mara Selvini-Palazzoli (Selvini,1988) p. 243	"Positive Connotation"*: The therapist ascribes a meaning to the symptom that is inspired by the altruistic goal of preserving the cohesion of the family.	Useful because it allows therapist access to system by not blaming symptomatic person. Highlights symptom's homeostatic function and can offer alternative meaning and, therefore, different remedial action.
p. 305	"Odd Days and Even Days Prescription" The therapist suggests to parents of symptomatic child: "On odd days, mom handles problem in any way she sees fit, without interference from dad. On even days, dad pursues any course of action that he deems appropriate, also without comment from mom." The child is asked to note any infractions.	Useful for parents whose disagreement about a course of action seems to be preventing resolution of a child problem. Can be combined with observe task to note which days the problem is improved. Can also be used with individuals torn between two decisions or solutions.
Journal of Marital and Family Therapy (Selvini-Palazzoli, 1986) p.340	"The Invariant Prescription" The parents of a troubled child are told to keep the content of treatment secret and to note the reactions of others to the secret. Parents are given instructions to disappear for increasingly longer periods of time and to note the responses of child and others in a notebook for discussion with the therapist.	Highlights couple as a separate entity, and as hierarchically superior to child. Introduces a variety of opportunities for meaning revision. Developed as a research tool for schizophrenia.

(*The Work of Mara Selvini-Palazzoli* also includes other rituals and prescriptions.)

In Search of Solutions, O'Hanlon & Weiner-Davis (1989) p. 128	"Complaint Pattern Intervention": The therapist arranges for the client to alter the performance of the complaint in some small or insignificant	

	way. For example, cigarette smoker to put cigarettes in attic, matches in basement.	Altering the performance of the complaint alters the context, enabling revision of the problem experience.
p. 132	"Context Pattern Intervention": The therapist can alter the personal or interpersonal patterns surrounding or accompanying the complaint. For example, a person who binges on food may avoid going out with friends on the binging days. The binger is asked to see friends on binging days.	This intervention consists of altering patterns not directly involved in the performance of the complaint.
p. 137	"The Surprise Task—For Couples or Families"*: "Do at least one or two things that will surprise your parents (spouse). Don't tell them what it is. Parents, your job is to see if you can tell what it is he/she is doing. Don't compare notes."	This task introduces randomness and playfulness into patterns. It may change the context of their difficulty. What may have been a battle, may now have a "gamelike" quality. Enables exceptions to be noted and amplified.
p. 138	"The Generic Task": The therapist uses client language to design an intervention that sets up expectancy for change. For example, if a client wants more peace of mind, suggest "Keep track of what you are doing this week that gives you more peace of mind."	This task presupposes that desirable behaviors will occur in between therapy sessions. Vague clients return with their goals more clearly defined. Enables exceptions to be noted.
Overcoming Relationship Impasses (Duncan & Rock, 1991), p. 51	"Inviting What You Dread": The therapist encourages the individual worried about another person's negativism to accept, validate, and even ex-	Useful when one person is sad, depressed, or pessimistic and verbalizes it, while other person is distressed by the complaints. Inter-

aggerate the complaints, and to initiate conversation about the complaints.

rupts usual solutions of cheerleading and avoiding.

p. 63

"Quid Pro Quo"*: (1) Clients tell each other what they would like to see more of or less of (10 min); (2) both repeat lists; (3) each explains how he or she has contributed negatively to the relationship (5 min.); (4) clients prioritize lists; (5) negotiation of each item begins by specification of what first indication of item would look like; (6) person requesting item asked what *he or she* can do to permit or make easier the desired change; and (7) agreement on item and both encouraged to observe results.

Useful for clients having difficulty discussing problems and who want a facilitator (therapist) to help them communicate. Enables an opportunity for a revision experience.

p. 72

"Agree and Exaggerate"*: Therapist suggests to a criticized person: (1) agree in words, but not in action (don't change behavior); (2) don't explain or defend self; (3) exaggerate criticism in nonsarcastic way.

Useful for clients who feel controlled and manipulated by another's criticism. Enables disempowered person to take charge of own feelings as well as the interaction.

p. 86

"Constructive Payback"*: Client is encouraged to attach indirect negative (but harmless) consequence to the chronically irritating behavior of another person (e.g., lateness, forgetfulness, incompetence, etc.)

Indirectly discharges anger and may create conditions for different meanings to emerge. Useful for adolescents or spouses who persist in grossly inconsiderate behavior despite multiple requests for change. Is also fun and tends to loosen things up.

p. 97 | Strategy for "Sexual Frequency": The therapist suggests to a sexually frustrated partner: (1) Remove all pressure and accompany by nonsexual affection; (2) spend time together in mutually enjoyable, nonsexual activities; (3) reduce sexual availability (not spitefully). | The basic strategy is to remove all pressure for sex, direct and indirect (no initiation of sex or conversations about it, no sexy clothes, no romantic rendezvous). Allows pressured spouse the space to feel sexual feelings.

p. 121 | "Giving Up Power To Gain Effectiveness"*: The therapist encourages clients to "give up" the fight verbally, but still be free to do whatever they behaviorally. | This is useful in a relationship in which there is an ongoing power struggle.

Overcoming Relationship Impasses also includes strategies for affairs, lack of communication, power disparities, and other relationship problems.

Appendix B

Quick Reference for Repeated Case Examples

THROUGHOUT this volume, we follow several clients through the treatment process. All identifying information has been altered. To facilitate the task of remembering the continuing case examples, this quick reference provides a brief description and a page number where a more detailed description is provided.

Case	Presenting problem/ identifying information	Interventions
Lynn, p. 25	9-year-old daughter's unhappiness and irritability viewed as signs of genetic depression.	Mother asked to encourage daughter's negative expressions, validate them, and exaggerate them.
Anita, p. 26	Suicide attempt and subsequent hospitalization; seemed enslaved by diagnosis of Borderline Personality Disorder.	Therapist asked what if the diagnosis was inaccurate; suggested a different one.
Joe, p. 48	Arrested for disturbing the peace; believed he was messenger from God having difficulty spreading His Word.	Because of the power of the message, the therapist suggested that Joe convey God's Word in subtle, yet important, ways.
Mark, p. 55	Depression, inability to concentrate; 38-year-old student with his whole life on the line.	Mark asked to observe differences between when he was able to concentrate and when he was not; Mark was also asked to

		perform an "ordeal" regarding his sleeping problem.
Richard, p. 72	Discovered that wife had an affair, no one believed him; presented as hostile and agitated.	Therapist suggested that he was proving his wife right, and that maybe returning to work and spending positive time with kids might help counter her accusations about his sanity.
Eric, Terry, & Michelle, p. 78	Initial presentation was suicidal adolescent; wanted second opinion, evolved into wanting help with Michelle's verbal abusiveness of Terry.	Therapist negotiated no-suicide contract and suggested an observe task; therapist suggested "giving up power" and "constructive payback."
Sandra, p. 80	Depression falling out of the blue; unfolded as related to husband's erectile difficulties.	Therapist suggested that the depression and impotence problem protected the marriage.
Mary, p. 98	Marital problem related to husband's recent avoidance of home; wanted to save marriage.	Therapist suggested the Mary make herself less available to her husband.
Janice, p. 102	Fear of flying; believed fears to be overreaction.	Therapist suggested a symptom prescription, taught a relaxation exercise, and suggested an airport rating task.
Alice, David, & Jill, p. 142	Jill cut her wrists and threatened suicide; emotional outbursts identified her as different from her sisters.	Asked parents to note the things they observed in Jill that they would like to see continue. Parents' ascriptions of new meanings were empowered by the therapist.

Monte, p. 143	High anxiety, panic attacks; feared that he would wind up like his father, hopelessly mentally ill.	Therapist suggested a symptom prescription. Monte's ascriptions of new meanings were empowered by the therapist.
Ted, p. 155	Panic attacks; wanted to know options for treatment because of familiarity with different modalities from a course he had taken.	Therapist ascribed a smorgasbord of meanings from a variety of approaches and then suggested a symptom prescription.
Joan, p. 159	Drinking problem; believed that she was unable to stop drinking because her mother had damaged her emotionally.	Therapist ascribed the meaning of showing respect to Joan's continued drinking.
Hal, p. 163	Depression, suicidal thinking; felt like a loser about his career and resented his father's control.	Therapist suggested "dangers of improvement" and suggested the depression rating and predicting task. Hal's new meanings were empowered by the therapist.

☒ Index